ARLINE AND JOHN LIGGETT

The Tyranny of Beauty

LONDON
VICTOR GOLLANCZ LTD
1989

Also by John Liggett
THE HUMAN FACE

First published in Great Britain in 1989
by Victor Gollancz Ltd
14 Henrietta Street, London WC2E 8QJ

© Arline and John Liggett 1989

British Library Cataloguing in Publication Data
Liggett, Arline
    The tyranny of beauty.
    1. Beauty. Sociological perspectives
    I. Title   II. Liggett, John
    302.5

ISBN 0-575-04430-6

Photoset by Rowland Phototypesetting Ltd, Bury St Edmunds, Suffolk
Printed in Singapore for Imago

THE TYRANNY OF BEAUTY

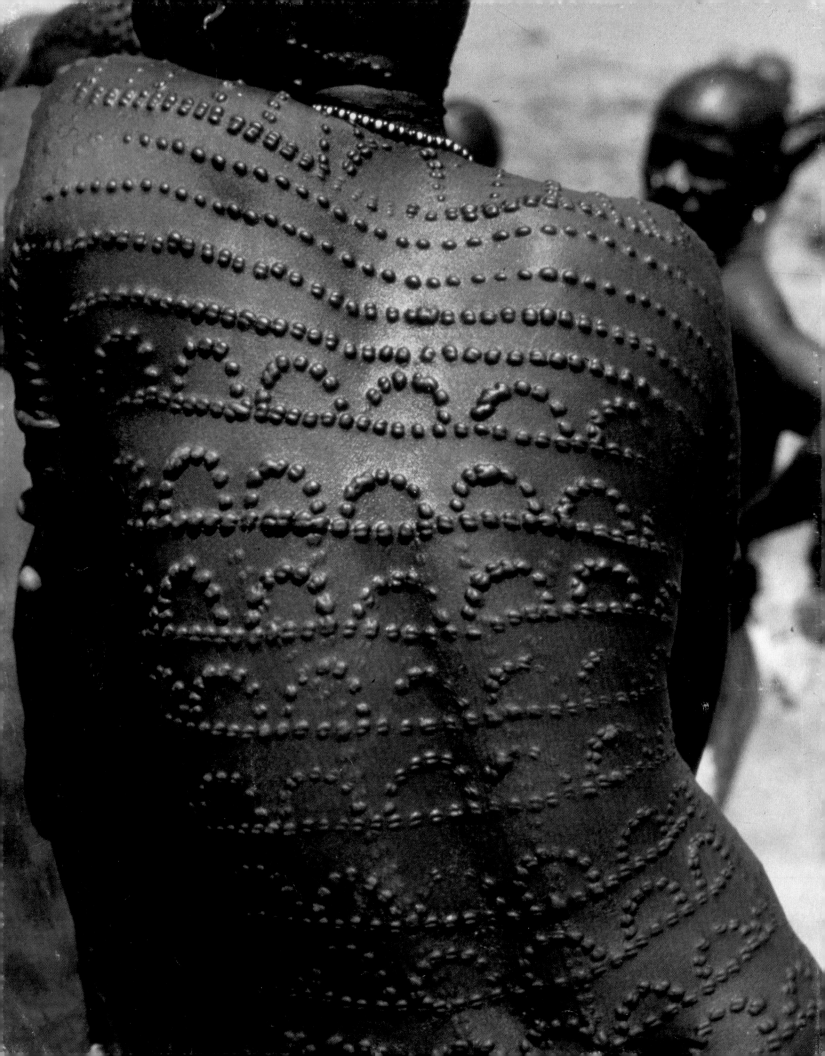

TO SPENCER

FRONTISPIECE : As well as enhancing appearance, elaborate body scarring can also tell who you are and what you are

OVERLEAF, PAGES 8 / 9 : A way of stretching the neck shown in a caricature of a school of beauty, c. 1800

ACKNOWLEDGEMENTS

The writers gratefully acknowledge the assistance of the Wellcome Museum of the History of Medicine, European Research Consultants International, The Trading Standards Safety Officer, Cardiff, and Gareth Jenkins, Features Editor of the *Western Mail*. Thanks are due for valuable technical advice to Kenneth Bevan and to Anthony Davidson and colleagues of the Cardiff Library for their tireless research and to Eric, John, Alma, Joan, Jane, Mary, Deryck, Christine and Lynda for their wise and helpful discussions. A special debt of gratitude is owed to Elfreda Powell of Gollancz for her skilled help, unfailingly good advice, and cheerful encouragement.

A.L. & J.L.
January 1989

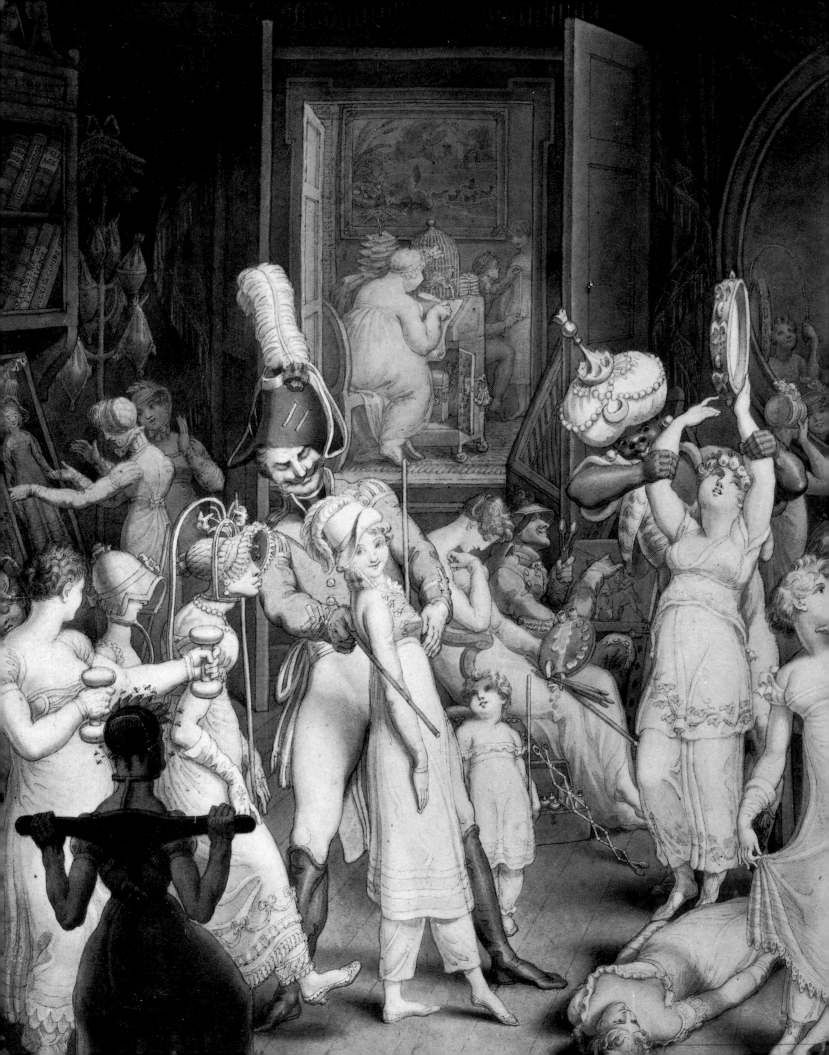

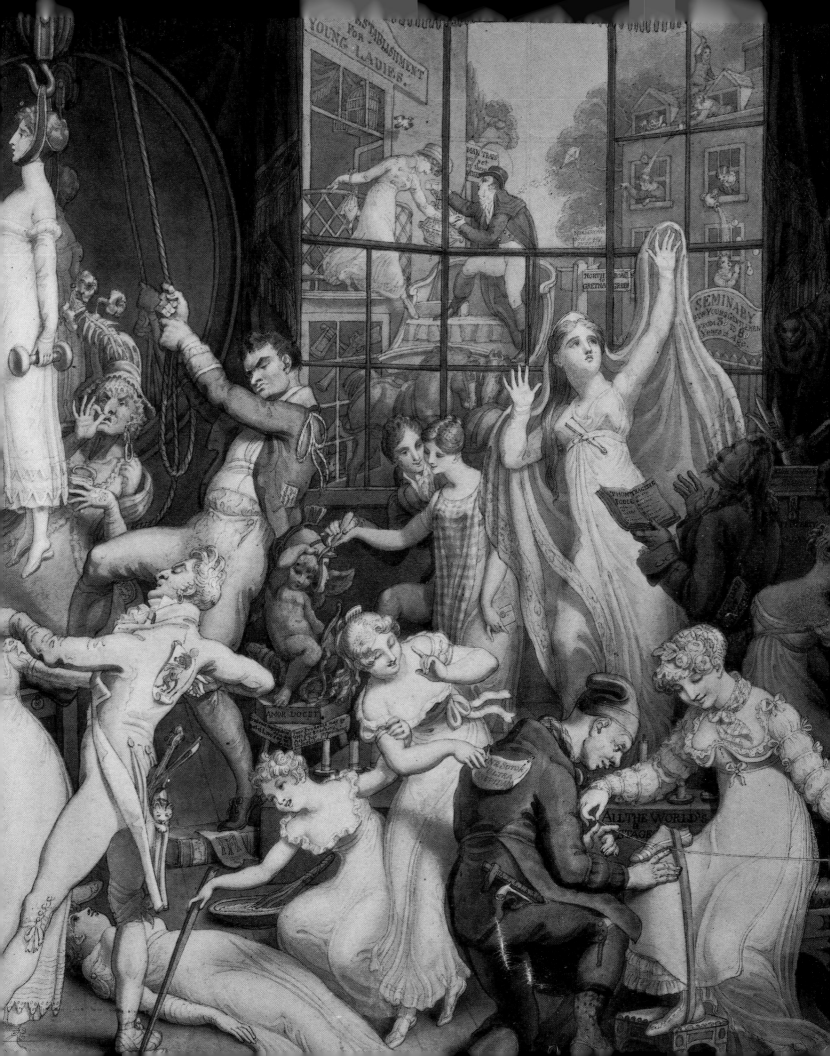

CONTENTS

CONTENTS

INTRODUCTION

For as long as history can trace, men and women have rushed eagerly into beautifying routines of an agony which – in any other context – would be described as 'torture'. No aspect of the human body has been spared. The battle has been waged, not simply to enhance the appearance, but also to transform it quite radically, and often with scant regard for the cost.

To achieve an ideal, women have broken their feet, lost their hair, poisoned their skins with lead – even died in their search for beauty. Crocodile dung and pigeon's pellets have been pasted on to faces: lizards have been boiled, lemons squeezed and livestock slaughtered for their magical parts, all in the desperate cause of self-improvement. An elderly romantic novelist, renowned for her youthful looks, has recently admitted to a home-made face-lift relying on Elastoplast and string.

Today, cosmetic surgery creates beauty to order. Some surgeons, confident of their personal trade-mark, boast they can identify at a glance which bosoms are 'theirs', and which someone else's. And not just bosoms are re-structured; hips, bottoms, thighs, chins, cheekbones, noses, mouths and hair might well all be credited to this or that plastic surgeon or cosmetician. Women can now be man-made and then – if they are truly desperate – be maintained in a perpetually youthful condition by regular cocktails of the macerated foetuses of unborn animals.

Men have been equally vain. The daily ritual of the eighty-year-old Maréchal de Richelieu included having the loose skin of his face pulled up and then pinned to a pad which he kept tucked under his thinning hair. Men in the sixteenth century often sported a flamboyant cod-piece so grotesquely accommodating that there was usually space for knick-knacks and a toffee or two in it. But at least they had freedom to move. Which is more than can be said for those twentieth-century men who have risked temporary sterility by confining themselves within the tightest of jeans in order to exhibit an extravagant masculinity.

Nowadays, to improve their looks, males have their faces surgically altered. Some dye their hair. Some have their genitals tattooed. Some paint their faces, others take drugs to change the colour of their skin. Many professional men say they need to look young to keep their jobs in a competitive world. Higher standards of performance are demanded both in bedroom and in boardroom. Losing weight has become all-important but there are penalties to be paid; in the first half of 1988 alone, 25,000 men were known to have developed anorexia nervosa. And now, psychological problems are on the increase; men are becoming afflicted with sudden impotence. And this has driven some of them to restorative injections sometimes so excessively effective that surgical intervention has been required to quieten them down. The situation is not without its lighter side. Men smile wryly about the use of inflatable prosthetic devices serviced by a pump mechanism lodged in the scrotum.

There have been some disarming attempts at togetherness in the search for beauty. Women have looked to men for help and vice-versa. Sex they always knew was good for beauty. But there have been other touching alliances too. In the seventeenth century interdependency reached its peak when women were recommended to bathe in male urine, a substance much prized as 'highly beneficial and greatly beautifying'. In the United States today, there are flourishing beauty clinics employing 'urine therapy' and plenty of women quaff their own urine for health and beauty.

Yet though men have castigated and women have occasionally complained, at no time in history have they ever seriously questioned why they continue to go to such lengths in order to change their bodies.

This book takes a closer look at some of the more outrageous attempts at beautification in ancient as well as modern times – at the bizarre efforts of the fops and the dandies – the hilarious antics of the courtesans, queens and housewives of history – as well as the more technologically sophisticated experiments of their modern counterparts.

What emerges is an extraordinary catalogue of behaviour, sometimes tragic, but frequently comic, which throws much light on one of the more mysterious corners of human psychology – the varied, often unsuspected motives underlying the eternal pursuit of beauty.

1. STARVING FOR STYLE

They say that nobody loves you if you are fat . . . and especially if you are a woman. Indeed, in the western world, the outsize woman has rarely been popular. Leading couture houses do not cater for her. Creative stylists find little inspiration in meeting her aesthetic needs. And the brutal truth is not kept from her. Top American designer Calvin Klein did not mince his words: 'I don't want women bigger than a size 12 wearing my clothes.'

Slimness is ceaselessly, almost monotonously equated with beauty. In the fantasy world of magazine, film, and popular novel, the female form which is identified with love, wealth, success, sexuality, happiness is almost always slim. In the real world too, few females see themselves as thin enough to be really beautiful. They hanker for the pared-down lines of models and actresses who stare from magazine pages with the waif-like look of the under-nourished, or with the superior glare of remote creatures who have risen above the coarse habit of eating.

Women in the public eye are especially nervous. Opera singers, in particular, have often had a hard struggle with the problems of appearing frail and delicate in spite of their own massive bulk (mysteriously allied to their nightingale voice). The soprano Marie Wilt, described by one expert in the early 1900s as having 'the finest voice I have ever heard', was known in Vienna as the 'Imperial Elephant'. Unhappily at the age of fifty-eight, she fell disastrously in love with a younger man who – because of her size – found it impossible to return her love. In despair, she threw herself from a fourth-floor window.

THINNER AND THINNER

Maria Callas too was deeply conscious of her hefty figure which she truly felt to be the only remaining deterrent to a great career. She began reducing her weight in the spring of 1953. By April 1954, she had lost nearly sixty-two pounds – more than half a hundred-weight of too, too solid flesh. But she kept the secret of her diet to herself: 'I had a tapeworm and I no longer have it,' was all she was prepared to reveal. It seems likely that she was speaking factually. A tapeworm-cyst-pill had already been marketed in the 1930s before this later one which deliberately introduced a tapeworm into the system, together with instructions on how to remove it, hopefully before too much toxic damage had occurred.

Many stars from stage and screen have kept flabbiness at bay at enormous personal cost. Joan Crawford lived for a time on nothing but crackers and mustard. The actress Diana Wynyard died from slimming. Judy Garland, at the age of fourteen, worked herself to exhaustion on a diet of chicken soup, amphetamines and sleeping tablets.

OPPOSITE : Slimness is ceaselessly, almost monotonously, equated with beauty

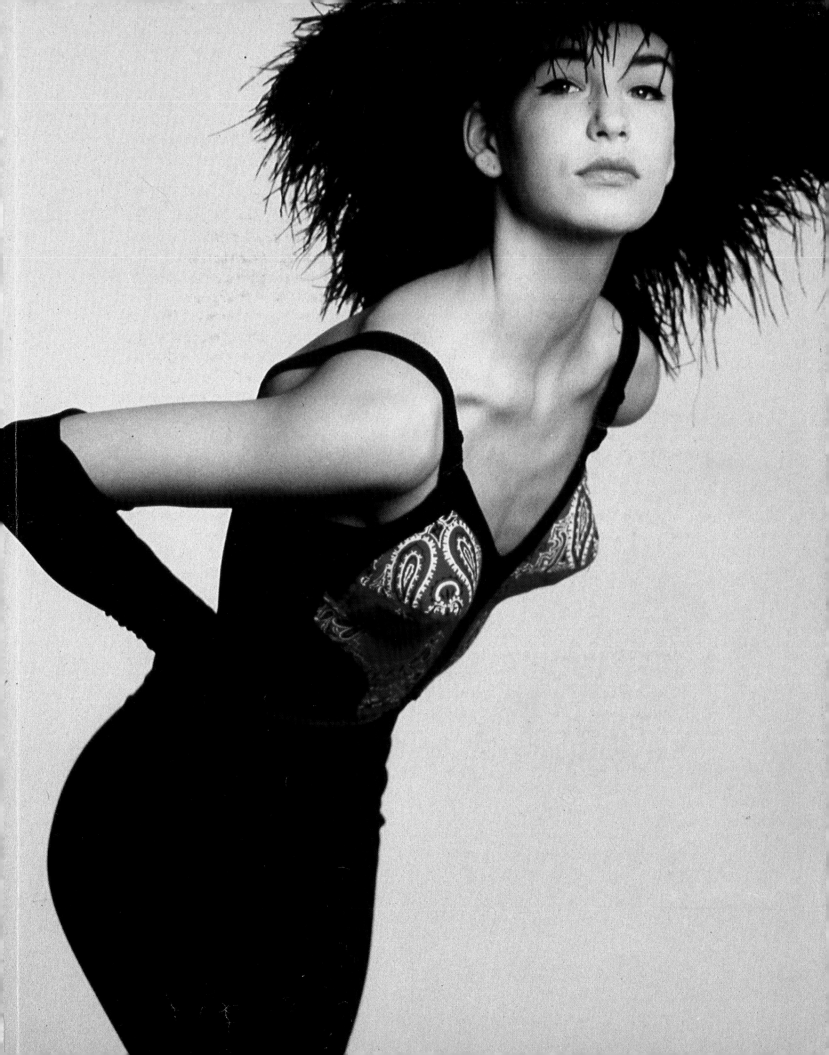

Books on how to lose weight are produced *ad nauseam*, and are snapped up by insatiable searchers-after-leanness. Any new title has a good chance of appearing in the best-seller columns: books such as Rosemary Conley's 'Hip and Thigh Diet'. Ms Conley had ingeniously detected a gap in a seemingly already saturated market – the need for 'spot-reducing'. Under the Conley regime, women suffering from 'uneven weight distribution' are encouraged to select the part they wish to reduce – say a thick waist – and told how to reduce this without sacrificing, say, the bosom.

Martin Katahn's 'Rotation Diet' has concentrated on the formidable and seemingly inevitable problem faced by most dieters – how to avoid putting on weight again, once a diet is halted. The body is very accommodating – it cuts back on its need for calories when it is given less food, but it is slow to re-adjust when more normal eating starts again. The sudden extra calories it receives are usually laid down as fat. Katahn's regime requires a diet of only three weeks' duration, in the first instance, during which time the average loss for women will be fourteen pounds (more for men). After these first twenty-one days a complete break for a week, or even a month is prescribed. In other words, the 'Rotation Diet' aims at never allowing the body to reduce its metabolic needs, thus doing away with any 'rebound' weight-gaining when normal eating begins again.

Other regimes are attractive because they provide complete menus, with calorie and fibre content meticulously worked out. Audrey Eyton's 'F-Plan Diet' and 'Easier F-Plan Diet' give the weary dieter ready-made meal suggestions – precisely what to eat for breakfast, lunch and supper, down to the last shake of salt and spoonful of sugar.

But a great many diets have been controversial and have caused alarm in nutritionist circles. Take an adapted version of the 'Mayo Clinic Diet' which was recently circulating in London and which confidently insists, 'It is important to eat nine eggs the first day'. Totting up the total number of eggs permitted in just two weeks revealed an astonishing total of between fifty-six and fifty-eight eggs. Yet the medical view of eggs is solidly against a high intake of cholesterol. The Royal College of Physicians recommends no more than three eggs a week if we are to avoid heart disease.

A new 'American Fruit Diet' (in Harvey and Marilyn Diamond's *Fit For Life*) topped the New York best-seller list for forty weeks in 1987, but was described by Vincent Marks, Professor of Biochemistry at Surrey University, as 'a disaster for young people and a catastrophe for pregnant women and their babies'. 'When I read it,' he says, 'I thought it must be a spoof. The idea that young people might take it seriously is intensely horrifying.'

On the other hand, lovers of ice-cream can take heart. Dr Neil Solomon, a diet expert and former Assistant Professor of Psychiatry at Johns Hopkins School of Medicine in Baltimore, USA, points out that ice-cream satisfies the clamouring appetite for about two to three hours (better, for example, than chocolate which raises the blood sugar more rapidly but only quietens the hunger pangs for half an hour or so). 'The Ice-Cream Diet'

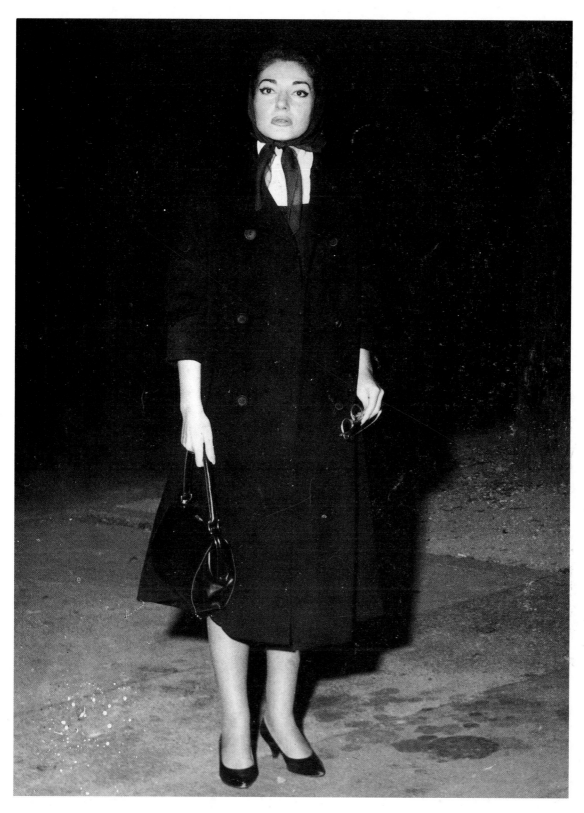

Maria Callas: 'I had a tapeworm and I no longer have it'

recommends a general diet of 1,030 calories a day, with a single level tablespoonful of ice-cream taken every two hours.

American psychologist Gayle Black focuses on idiosyncrasy. She believes that most diets are capable of working – it's the dieters who falter. In 'The Sun Sign Diet' Ms Black explains the mysterious astrological influences we receive from the stars and the rotation of the planets. Pisceans, for example, must come to terms with the fact that they are 'emotional eaters'.

The 'Herbalife Diet', which by 1984 had 20,000 followers in Britain, began in America in early 1980 but was rated 'a bad way to try to slim' by Oliver Gillie, then medical correspondent of *The Sunday Times*. It could, he believed, cause the body's metabolism to become unbalanced and produce 'abnormal quantities of nitrogen wastes which have to be eliminated through the kidneys in the urine' – a serious problem for the many people who have poor or indifferent kidneys.

But no diet has caused such a furore as Alan Howard's 'Cambridge Diet', and the American 'Liquid Protein Diet.'

The 'Cambridge Diet' offers for sale soups, milk-shakes and desserts, each portion rated at 110 calories; three portions a day to be consumed. Eight years of research are said to have gone into the diet's creation, with routine tests for safety, spread over three years. But when it was introduced into the United States in the spring of 1980 it immediately suffered setbacks. The US Government halted sales, saying that advertised claims were false. Shortly afterwards, consent for sales was given, providing certain warnings were put on the cans.

But the diet seemed doomed to misfortune. Six deaths occurred coincidentally in people taking the 'Cambridge Diet' and it was rigorously investigated by the FDA (Food and Drug Administration). The outcome was that a relationship between cause of death and the 'Cambridge Diet' could not be proved or disproved.

And then in mid-1982 – as its founder regretfully but frankly points out in his book *The Cambridge Diet* – salmonella was found in a few cans of the diet and customers were asked to return certain dated tins. The diet is now marketed in sachets, instead of tins. Their latest pamphlet (at the time of writing) warns of possible minor side-effects associated with many weight loss programmes: headaches, mild dizziness, constipation, diarrhoea, nausea, irritability and dryness of the skin.

Criticism of the 'Cambridge Diet' was concerned in the main with its low-calorie content, perhaps best summed up by Dr Thomas A. Wadden of the University of Pennsylvania: 'The prolonged use of very low calorie diets clearly results in large losses of lean body mass in some persons. Perhaps the greatest risk in this area is that even small losses could have unfortunate consequences if they were to occur from critical organs, such as the heart.'

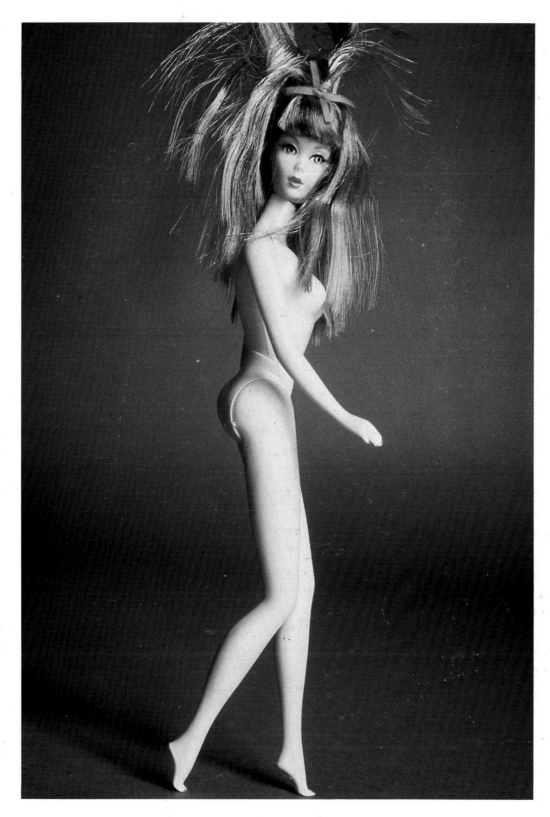

The etiolated shape of the 'Ideal Woman'?

And the diet also had problems with its marketing. In the United States, it had been launched by entrepreneurs, Jack and Eileen Feather, who sold it by mail order. The Feathers had no inhibitions about exploiting the prestigious Cambridge image. Cans of the produce bore a brash logo with – to the outrage of many indignant Fellows – a drawing of the gate of Trinity College Cambridge. In fact, the logo seemed to start a trend for products with an academic cachet. All at once there was the 'Oxford Diet', the 'Eton Diet' and, more comprehensively, the 'University Diet'.

Unfortunately, the creative Jack Feather had himself invented a number of devices for slimming – the 'Astro Trimmer' for waist and tummy, the 'Sauna Belt' and others, including a 'Mark Eden Bust Developer' designed to allow women to develop their busts at the same time as slimming other, less desirably bulky parts. In 1982 a Grand Jury indicted the Feathers for mail order malpractice. The marketing of the bust developer and the sauna devices ceased. And, inevitably, some of the opprobrium reflected on the 'Cambridge Diet' which the Feathers were also marketing.

At this time, too, American memories were still fresh from the scandal of the 'Liquid Protein Deaths'. In the 1970s, George Blackburn, a Harvard professor, promoted his so-called 'Protein-sparing Modified Fast'. It involved taking vitamin and mineral tablets with a quarter of a pound of lean steak every day. At about the same time a research chemist discovered a chemical process for making protein from cowhide rendered soluble in water. This cowhide protein was of poor quality and deficient in many important amino-acids but it had the advantage of being much cheaper than steak – so it was sweetened with saccharine, flavoured with cherry and marketed as 'Liquid Protein Diet'. It never underwent rigorous clinical testing but was successfully marketed under as many as fifty different brand names, and it sold well.

By the end of 1978, however, the American FDA were becoming concerned about deaths following its use. Out of fifty reports, seventeen were clearly linked to 'Liquid Protein Diet'. Death was said to be caused by the heart's developing abnormal rhythms for which there was no effective treatment. Once admitted to hospital, these dysrhythmic patients failed to respond to any of the known medical treatments and eventually died. Autopsies revealed severe degeneration of the heart muscle.

In 1984, the FDA created new regulations: all preparations having more than 50% of their total calories derived from protein or liquid protein and containing fewer than 400 calories were required to carry the following warning: 'These preparations may cause serious illness or death.' In his book of 1985 defending the 'Cambridge Diet', Alan Howard was quick to point out that the FDA decided that this warning was not necessary in the case of the 'Cambridge Diet'.

But dieting to lose weight is not always necessary, say the promoters of alternative methods. How about a nice cup of tea instead? At first glance, not a bad idea, especially when the tea is apparently endorsed by the Duchess of York. Such was the boast of 'Bai Lin Tea', together with a promise that it would 'dissolve away the pounds'. 900,000 packets were sold in Britain for a total of four and a half million pounds. But alas, the product – supposedly based on an ancient Chinese recipe – turned out to be nothing more than ordinary China tea, and claims of the Duchess's endorsement were dismissed by Warwick Crown Court in June 1988, as 'bogus'.

For those who want to slim, indulging in a good fidget sounds a whole lot simpler as well as being a good deal less expensive. And according to recent research it might even be just as effective. Scientists measuring the number of calories lost by scratching and twitching have discovered that big-time fidgets use up energy which is equal to a three-mile run every day.

The human mind is incredibly fertile when it comes to creating new ideas for losing weight. Yet there is nothing at all new about slimming. In the fourteenth century, the Queen of France, Isabeau of Bavaria, was one of the earliest fanatics to go on record. She stayed for hours in special sweating rooms with 'cupping glasses' pressed to her body to squeeze away the fat.

A later recipe in 1665, entitled 'To Reduce the body that is too fat to a mean and handsome proportion', favoured both sweating, purging and bleeding: 'Rise early in the mornings and use some violent exercise to sweat often. It is good to bleed largely, twice a year, the right arm in the spring, the left in the autumn; purge the body in those seasons with strong physic.'

As for those specific parts of the body which persisted in bulging and causing displeasure, they should have their food supply cut off with 'ligaments to bind those passages where the member is supplied with nourishment'.

It is only in the West that obesity is undesirable: in today's famine-racked world there are many countries where attitudes to plumpness are very different. In Bangwa in the Cameroons, for example, and in many other parts of Africa, fatness brings prestige. Only the upper-class can afford to eat well; a plump woman's family must therefore be assumed to be well-to-do. And with any luck, the rich, plump woman will continue to be plump throughout her life. Not so the poor women who must work on the land for a living. For such women, the opportunity to become so desirably fat occurs just once in their lives. Before marriage they will be housed in a special, fattening-up room where they will be made to eat for seven to nine weeks, and where their bodies will grow, and their breasts will swell. But, alas, this bliss is shortlived. After marriage, it is back to the fields and for the rest of their lives little more than a survival diet.

In North Africa, in order to ensure their desirability in the marriage market, young girls are fattened with buttermilk, porridge and plenty of bread. And during the three weeks immediately before the wedding, they are force-fed with supplementary pellets of bread.

In many parts of East Africa, wealthy wives are obliged to drink immense quantities of milk. They become so fat that observers have said they can sometimes only crawl about on hands and knees.

THE BODY-BUILDERS

Europeans who wish to become bigger usually aim not for fat, but muscle. Every pound of muscle weight the body-builder can add to his or her weight will use up 50–100 calories a day. So the more muscle they put on, the more heartily Mr and Ms Universe can eat. Muscles are of double value – they have both dramatic effect and the ability to burn up calories.

But a perfectionistic approach to bodily beauty can come to dominate a man's life. Lee Harvey, Mr Olympia and four times Champion of Britain, constantly searches the mirror for signs of flaws – could the calves be bigger, the biceps more peaked? Hours of strenuous training go into the production of his superman body – and mental energy too: 'It's as if you're willing the muscle to superhuman contraction, and the body won't go where the mind has not gone first. I see myself sculpting my body, turning it into a work of art. So I'm not satisfied just to develop big arms – I want great arms, with every detail and proportion correct, something great artists like Michelangelo and Leonardo da Vinci would admire.'

For the committed muscle-man, new standards and ever more ambitious ideals to be achieved are created every day. Scores of specialist magazines cater for his needs. And hers too. For this is no longer a male preserve: women are just as dedicated.

Corinna Everson, who won the Ms Universe title in 1987 has pointed out that women have to put so much more effort into their appearance at Championship Shows, than do male competitors. 'First we have to fuss so much with our hair the week before the Show. Fixing my hair took about three hours the day of the Show. . . . Getting the right suit requires a week of excruciating fits and refits. Add another three hours for make-up and final suit-fit the day of the Show. Then too, we are subject to hormonal changes each month. That can add 3lbs of water and a special kind of irritability. With all that, women have to go through the same dieting, the same hard training and one heck of a lot more posing trials and tribulations.'

For both men and women the search for perfection means unending exercises, the consumption of canthaxanthin to produce the obligatory tan, often enough, other drugs besides. The use of anabolic steroids began around 1952 at the time of the Helsinki Olympic Games. At first it was only competitive body-builders who used them, but by 1980 it had become standard practice, deplored by many. Nowadays, diuretics have become popular aids for removing water from the system; cocaine is used to keep athletes up to standard as energy levels drop; masking agents are employed to camouflage urine samples which might be taken; steroid-induced acne is common.

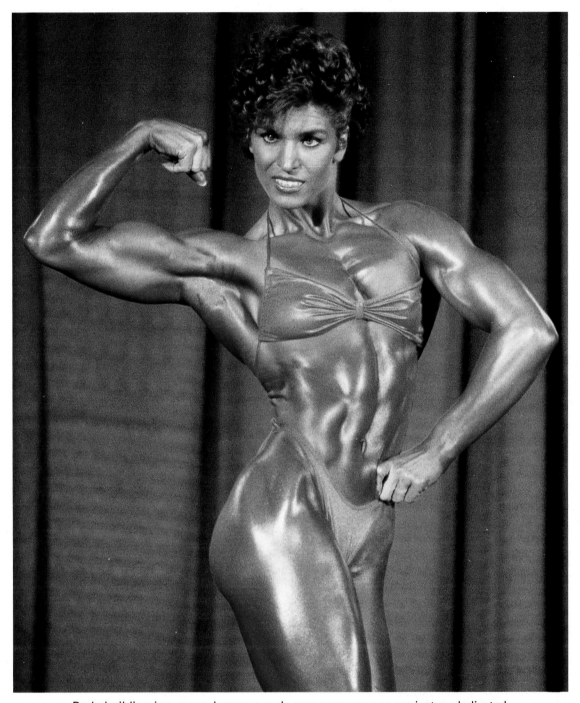

Body building is now no longer a male preserve: women are just as dedicated

The temptation to achieve more seems irresistible. Body-builders can soon become 'hooked' on drugs. And yet, as Jeff Everson says: 'The vast majority don't like it and only do it to keep up with the Joneses.'

FAT-REMOVERS

Plenty of women have looked to the sort of technology employed in body-building, but for just the opposite reason – to help them cut down, rather than build up, their size.

Three types of machine – all originating in France – have enjoyed some popularity. The 'Oxlender 2000' is a kind of space-ship module within which a woman, or man, is invited to lie, waiting to be sprayed with water, steam, oxygen, ozone and herbal oils – all intended to rejuvenate tissues, accelerate metabolism, and generally tone and slim the body.

The 'Oxlender's' sister model, the 'Physiomex', promises to improve circulation and remove undesirable fat. It resembles a blood-pressure measuring-cuff and uses an inflatable rubber hose to squeeze the legs and any other areas showing signs of flabbiness. But there are dangers; a reporter from the *The Sunday Times* tried out the 'Physiomex' and a large swelling to the elbow appeared, caused by the breaking of a small blood vessel.

Some beauty salons. advertise the 'Dyna Gym' exercising machine. This piece of equipment looks rather like a sliding ironing-board on a ladder. Strapped to it, those who feel they are overweight can shunt themselves energetically backwards and forwards, burning up calories as fast as their arms can take them.

Another machine, the 'Mediaphore', uses electrical impulses to encourage absorption of a special 'slimming' substance called Cellulium into the tissues.

But if none of these devices appeals, then there is always the 'Biofeedback Belt', the invention of a psychologist who has put learning theories to work. A friendly enough looking gadget, rather like a car's safety belt, the Biofeedback Belt aims at encouraging posture control and reducing abdominal flabbiness. All the owner has to do is wear it. But too much relaxing . . . and the Biofeedback becomes a scold. Every time the wearer's tummy slips out of place, it squeaks in a nasty, nagging manner, reminding her to 'pull herself together'.

A quite different technique has become known as 'a clip on the ear'. With a special gun a doctor shoots a surgical staple into the slimmer's ear close to an appropriate acupuncture point. Whenever there is a craving for food, all the slimmer has to do is take hold of the staple and wiggle it.

The French have delved deeply into the anatomy of fatness and have concluded that much of the trouble arises from waterlogging of the body's cells. This, they say, creates cellulite – masses of hard, grainy nodules which stubbornly resist exercise and diet. So French clinics and salons offer a variety of hot poultices, paraffin wax packs, radioactive mud and impressive-looking machinery which – for a price – will judder and shake the cellulite out of any stricken individual. Alternatively – since even after this strenuous opposition, cellulite will determinedly creep back – a more permanent cure is sometimes tried. Three weeks of injections using an enzyme solution, with the help of a diuretic, are designed to break down swollen tissue and chase away unwanted toxins and fluids. The

British view of cellulite is more dismissive: Dr Miriam Stoppard says that cellulite is an invented name for something which does not exist.

'Ionisation' is yet another system employed in French salons. For this, the doctor will scrutinise the victim, weighing up the hills and dales of her body, rather in the manner of the head of the family preparing to carve the Sunday roast and wondering which bit to tackle first. Having decided on the portions to be annihilated, he straps specially impregnated pads to the offending parts. He then shoots a galvanic current through them to draw from the pads enzymes which then bombard the stubborn cellulite to disperse it.

One of the most dramatic methods guarantees to siphon away half a stone of fat in a single session, and in specific places too. Described as 'suction lipectomy' or 'liposuction' but more irreverently known as the 'slurp technique', this has proved surprisingly popular among women who feel their thighs look too heavy for today's tight jeans. But if the skin is inelastic – or if too much fat is taken – what to do with the loose skin left behind can be a problem. Still, the mottled, sagging flesh which frequently follows the removal of so much fat seems not to deter most women. More important is the contour of the covered leg.

GOING TO EXTREMES

In days gone by people tried to remove fat, often by exercise alone. Cecil Beaton tells of his Auntie Jessie who, when on holiday, used to put on a rubber corset and then played strenuous games of tennis until sweat 'poured in cascades from her head'.

Nowadays in the late 1980s, less exertion is called for. Women can give themselves up to a 'personalised sauna' – little more than a plastic mackintosh they can climb into – to sweat away unwanted pounds.

There are, of course, many other methods for reducing – not all of them healthy. Amphetamine drugs will suppress the appetite, but the effect is short-lived and the side-effects undesirable. The appetite inevitably returns, and the temptation then is to increase the dosage. And so begins a disabling dependency. Big doses cause attacks of panic, confusion and hallucinations.

Appetite may be controlled more safely by taking tablets or biscuits containing methyl-cellulose. These reduce the appetite by absorbing water from the stomach. They swell, giving a temporarily 'full' feeling. But in October 1988 suspect tablets containing guar-gum glucomannan galactomannan, sometimes sold as flakes or granules with added vitamins, were declared dangerous and under threat of being banned for sale by the government. Instead of expanding in the stomach they were swelling in the gullet and necessitating emergency surgery. One fifty-nine-year-old Australian spent two months in hospital suffering from a ruptured oesophagus after taking these slimming tablets.

And then there are laxatives, which cause water loss. Taken regularly, these can be dangerous since they may result in potassium and calcium depletion. If prolonged, such calcium loss can soften bone and inflame the bowel. And there is a much more serious hazard: potassium balance in the blood is a delicate business – an excess or a deficit can affect the heart.

There is yet another remedy, simple but effective. All it asks is that the jaws be stapled firmly together with wire. This will make the dangerous activity of eating impossible; at the same time, the victim may enjoy the luxury of feeling 'safe'. A surprising number of gallant, despairing people have engaged in this drastic and uncomfortable 'cure'.

Appalled by her twenty-stone figure, Barbara Quelch had her jaws wired, and kept them so for nine, weary months. She succeeded in getting her weight down to twelve and a half stone, but once her jaws were unwired she bounced back to her usual twenty stone. Yet in spite of this experience, which she describes as 'pretty horrific and very anti-social', Barbara Quelch remained determined to lose weight. She submitted herself to gastro-plasty, an operation which halves the size of the stomach and which therefore necessarily reduces the absorption and intake of food. For eight weeks after the operation she could take only fluids. No matter, she was delighted to find that she lost half a stone a week for the next five months. But, even months later, she was still being sick after meals, and has remained quite unable to eat certain foods such as meat and potatoes. Her main meals, she says, barely fill a saucer. Nevertheless, she has no regrets: 'I have always wanted to wear modern clothes and now I can go into a boutique and choose what I want rather than go for something just because it fits.'

The idea of resorting to surgery to deal with the problem of obesity originated in the United States. One of the earliest operations, the Jejuno-ileal bypass, attempted to short-circuit the small bowel and so prevent absorption of fats. But there were worrying side-effects – sometimes fatal. So a surgical attack on the stomach itself was tried, and in 1981 the first gastroplasty operation was performed at the Iowa City Hospital. In these early attempts, the stomach was stapled horizontally so that one half only could be used. In later operations, however, there was a refinement: it was found that partitioning the stomach vertically, rather than horizontally, reduced the distressing side-effects of nausea and vomiting.

Such extreme surgical measures can only be regarded as a last resort for people who are desperate. Benefits from these large operations may be short-lived because within three years the stomach may stretch again. The strictest discipline of eating only small amounts of food with no more than 500 calories a day must therefore be maintained for ever.

One very new, ingenious alternative to surgery is to introduce a 'balloon' of specially-prepared rubber into the stomach. The balloon is inflated and may be left in position for as long as three months. As many as 15,000 Americans have already had this treatment. But there are snags. First of all the balloons have to be replaced regularly – a decidedly

OPPOSITE : Marilyn Monroe, enema sessions before photo sessions

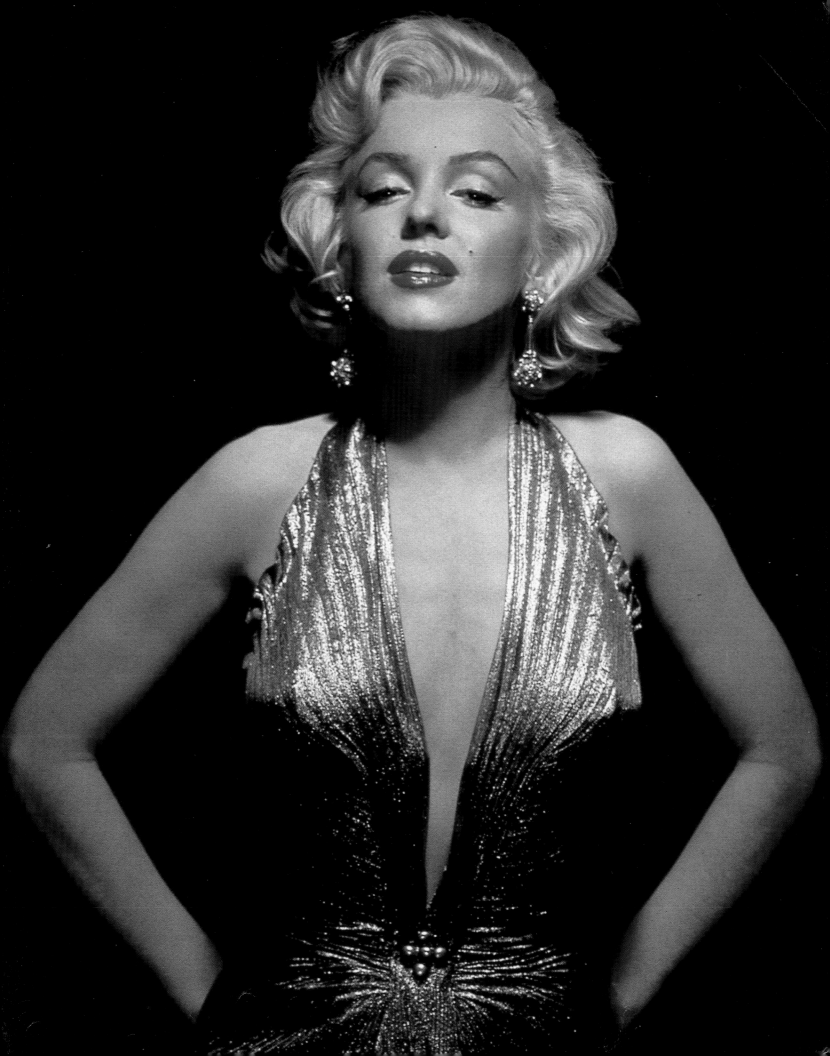

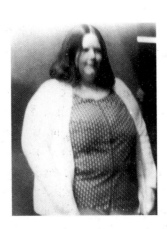

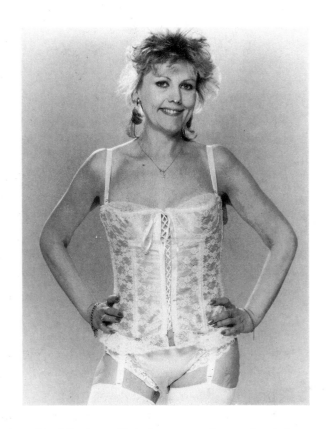

Shirley Rutherford, who once weighed 24 stone, has been whittled away to 8 by surgery: even her intestine has been shortened

unpleasant experience. Also, it is expensive. Dr Maclean Baird, a consultant physician, warns too that 'there is always the possibility of deflation and blockage of the bowels'. There can be no doubt, though, that the presence of these balloons does reduce hunger and therefore the desire to eat.

In the mid-Fifties, Marilyn Monroe is known to have taken frequent enemas. Among show business people this method was commonly used as an aid to instant weight loss, and especially for stars like Marilyn, anxious to flatten their stomachs before photographic sessions.

Women who are rich enough seem prepared to try anything to achieve the body they want. Actress Cher has had her tummy tightened, thighs reduced, bottom curvaceously reshaped, navel made more petite and 'girlish' – all topped off with no less than three breast lifts.

Shirley Rutherford, who once weighed twenty-four stone, has been whittled away to eight stone without dieting, but with almost everything snipped: thighs, knees, tummy, navel, breasts. And why stop at the outside? Even her intestine has been sliced almost all away to prevent food lingering there long enough to become fat.

To resist gross over-eating in the interests of good health is one thing, to become obsessed with the notion of losing weight is quite another, and especially when the body is already struggling at survival level. Yet today, more and more women, men – and most tragically of all – children are committed to the dangerous see-sawing business of binge-eating and starving. They are destined to become victims either of anorexia nervosa (the slimmers' disease) or bulimorexia (compulsive eating).

Fear of fat has developed into a serious complex that has far-reaching results. Desperate slimming regimes are changing lives, altering personalities and literally driving people to their deaths.

In 1976, *The British Journal of Psychiatry* reported that out of 12,000 schoolgirls over the age of sixteen, one in every 100 was suffering from anorexia nervosa. Recent case-histories and autobiographies reveal that the greatest spectre haunting the schoolgirl's life is the terror of becoming fat. There is clearly no place in a teenager's life for sturdy, developing limbs. Her fantasy world is peopled with the sylph-like, willowy-waisted women seen in television advertising. Her reality world of tight jeans affords no place for fat legs, plump stomachs or thick waists. Fat is disgusting. And so all over the Western world, girls with bodies like matchsticks starve themselves out of stark fear of ridicule.

The problem has now spread to younger children – some only eleven years old. Professor Bryan Lask at Great Ormond Street Hospital for Sick Children reported in 1988 a growing number of pre-teenage victims of anorexia. Whereas between the Sixties and early Eighties only about two cases a year were being treated, now there are three referrals a month. The anorexia pattern in children is similar to that in teenagers and adults, but among these young patients the percentage of males is higher than that among adults.

What causes it? Professor Lask and his team believe that increasing commercial pressure to be thin plays a part, though awareness of sexuality at an earlier age, family problems and a multiplicity of other complex psychological and social factors must also be considered.

The increase in the number of little boy anorexics is being mirrored now in young men who are also suffering. Career-conscious young professionals in their twenties are the hardest hit. 'I never used to see any business men, but I do now,' Dr Joan Gomex, a psychiatrist at the Gordon Hospital in London, has remarked. 'Two out of ten patients I see are men. They're very ambitious, they exercise non-stop and they don't want to be bothered with relationships. All they want is to look good.'

The word has got around that at job interviews thin men give the impression of vigour, energy and vitality. Today's ideal man created by advertising agencies is young, rich, handsome, successful and thin.

Barbara French, author of a book on bulimia, is quite clear that the media are largely responsible for the present spate of eating disorders, 'Thin people are always associated with the good life: expensive cars, beautiful jewellery, exotic holidays, all the glamorous things.'

One woman in Holland managed to gain admission to hospital to have her stomach pumped by claiming that she had taken an overdose of tranquillisers. She did this no less than seventy-five times. And she was only found out after being admitted to the Dutch National Poison Control Centre where it was discovered that although there were large quantities of recently-digested food in her stomach, there were no drugs. Her policy had been to satisfy her natural hunger with a substantial meal and then present herself for stomach-pumping.

Other women just waste away. In the UK between 1979 and 1984 there were 106 deaths from anorexia. Ballerina Janet French wasted to six stone and committed suicide. Lena Zavaroni is an anorexic still struggling to survive. Karen Carpenter in the USA died from anorexia. Louise Roche, author of *Glutton for Punishment*, at one time alternated binge-eating with starvation and amphetamines plus as many as thirty laxatives a day.

'It's worth it for the smug safety of the thinness of your body,' was the comment of one twenty-two-year-old secretary who had wasted away from ten to seven and a half stone. But there was a gnawing conflict. Though she was on the one hand experiencing a dreamy peace of mind, she also had bouts of shivering cold and bodily weariness. What should she do? Live the half-life of the anorexic with confidence and enjoyment and swinging moods of exhaustion and cold? Or should she eat and feel unloved, uncomfortable, vulnerable and appallingly depressed?

Susie Orbach suggests that it is modern male psychology which is playing a large part in the increase in anorexia. She says that it is males who promote thin bodies and encourage slimming because of 'a pervasive fear of women and a desire to package them safely into commodities'.

The weight problem for a woman today, however, may be much more subtle: it may consist in actually dealing with the challenging freedoms which have come with her newly found 'liberation'. One freedom is the freedom to be herself. But to experience this, she needs, first of all, to discover what her true self really is; she then has – as psychologist Dr Carl Rogers has explained – the infinitely harder problem of accepting the self she has discovered.

A few courageous women have recognised this and have made a start by trying first of all to accept what they see in the mirror. They have thrown away their slimming books and sometimes the weighing scales too. And they have decided to eat and exercise just when and how they please, whatever the outcome.

Nancy Roberts, author of *Breaking All the Rules – Feeling Good And Looking Great, No Matter What Your Size*, says: 'Being a large person is O.K. for me, and believing it has changed my life.' Food no longer dominates her waking life. She eats what she likes yet she neither loses weight nor gains it. 'This is me! This is it!' she says. She is Junoesque and completely guilt-free.

O P P O S I T E : 'When there's a bit of me I don't like, I change it.' Actress Cher has spent £24,000 on cosmetic surgery

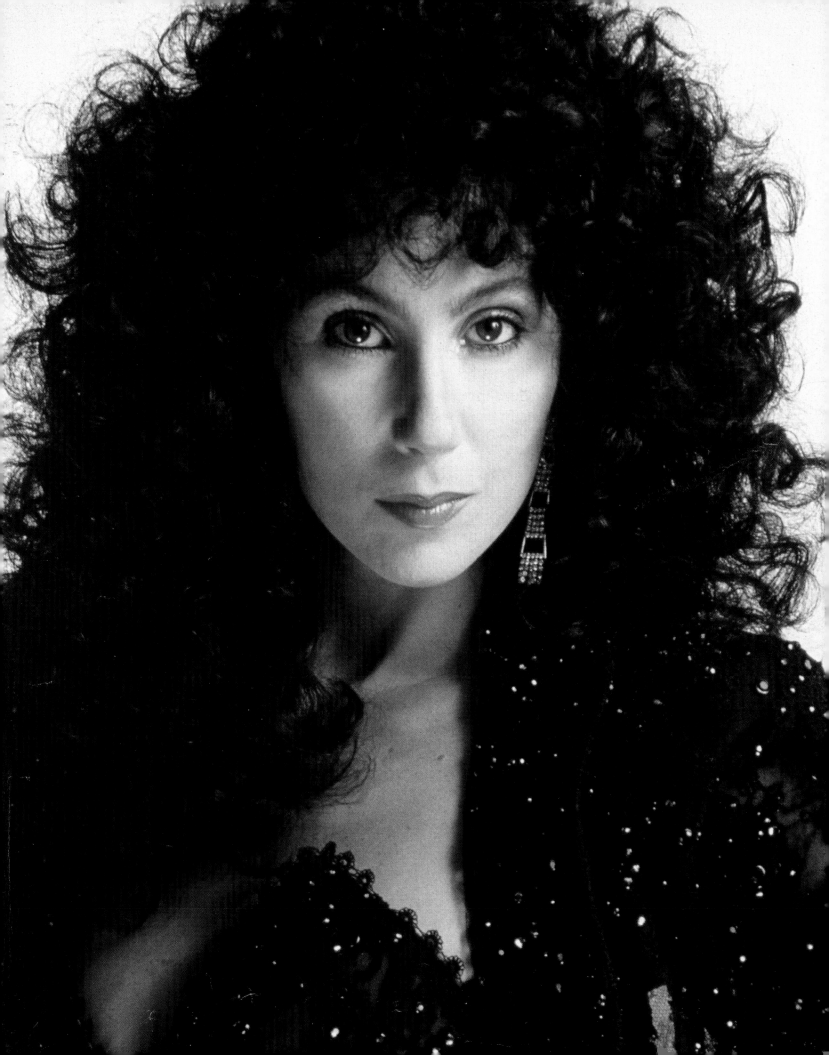

Other women have come to terms with their generous size, in a rather different way. Their natural bigness, they say, gives them a greater, all-embracing capacity to meet the emotional needs of others. With their motherliness – so evident in their ample frame – they can be less concerned with their own needs. They can accept instead the caring role of everyone's mother.

In many ways, woman's conflict with her body mirrors perfectly her ambivalent attitude to the stereotyped image of her place in society – that of help-mate, maternal provider, supportive aide – and, all too often, second-class citizen. Such a role has been thrust upon them, women feel, by the peculiar construction of their bodies. The limitations of their place in the world have come about through the restricting confines and specialised functions of the female form. Full breasts and rounded thighs are physical attributes which imply, if one begins to think about it, the responsibilities of bearing children and succouring man. This may in truth be a worthy enough destiny to fulfil. And some feel it is fulfilment enough. But others hanker after the privilege of discovering their true potential for themselves – to break free from the mould, to discover and, better still, fulfil all the additional talents and hidden capacities they might have. They want an unrestricted, unprejudiced opportunity to be creative intellectually, and not just physically.

In dieting and slimming they have unconsciously sought a device for emancipating themselves from their bodies – for wiping the slate clean, for finding their real selves, unfettered by bodily features with specialised functions they were never even consulted about.

It may be that when the really true self has been discovered, these same women will not wish to change themselves at all. But stripping the body of its blatantly feminine characteristics – paring it to the bone – will at least have demonstrated their determination to have some degree of freedom of choice, some say in their destiny.

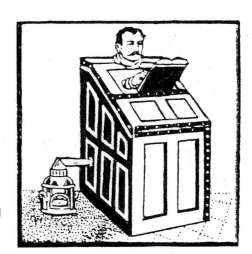

Foot's Bath Cabinet in which a man could enjoy his beauty treatment 'privately at home'

2. THE BEWILDERING BOSOM

It was a psychologist, the late Dr J. C. Flugel, who suggested that women's erotic charms were spread generously around her body and not – as with men – more specifically localised. He advanced the theory—endearing in its implications – that men find it difficult to drink in all of women's delights at once. A sip rather than a gulp is more desirable. Fashion's job, therefore, was to funnel woman's 'erotic capital' into just one part of the female form at a time. This year the bust – another year the legs, or the waist perhaps. Flugel called this the principle of 'shifting erogenous zones'. The triumphant fashion news in autumn 1988 was that 'bosoms are back'. To meet the requirements of this apocalyptic decision many models – insufficiently endowed – immediately opted for surgery to boost their assets.

RESTRAINING THE EXUBERANCY

In the 1920s, when it was the turn of the legs to be the focus of attention, the fashionable dress was waistless and breastless. Cecil Beaton described the ideal figure as 'of diminutive proportions and concave, instead of convex'. Colette added her definition, 'no more hip or belly or backside than a bottle of Rhine wine and above all, the chest of an ephebe'.

It was not the thing to be seen to have any breasts at all, so everything possible was done to make them disappear. A New York company – the Boyish Form Brassière Company – manufactured breast-constricting devices which, they promised, would 'give you that boy-like flat appearance'. The 'folded breast' was equally successful. To achieve this, the breast was doubled downwards and folded as close as possible against the ribs. An elastic binding might then be placed over the compressed bosom.

But there is nothing new in this idea. Tight breast bindings were popular in Ancient Greece and again in Chaucer's day in England. In Bavaria, it was one of the practices to strap wooden platters to girls' chests to compress their breasts. In Arabia, women were encouraged to cultivate tiny bosoms and were advised at all costs to 'restrain the exuberancy of overgrown breasts'. Circassians in Asia Minor went even further. They fastened young girls into leather garments for as long as seven years to give their figures greater symmetry. When the girls married it was the bridegroom's privilege to cut open the stitches in the leather with his knife. After that, the breasts were allowed to grow – if, indeed, they were still disposed to. What was cheerfully ignored was that many women became anaemic, frequently consumptive, and that a great many died. Yet the custom lasted well into the nineteenth century.

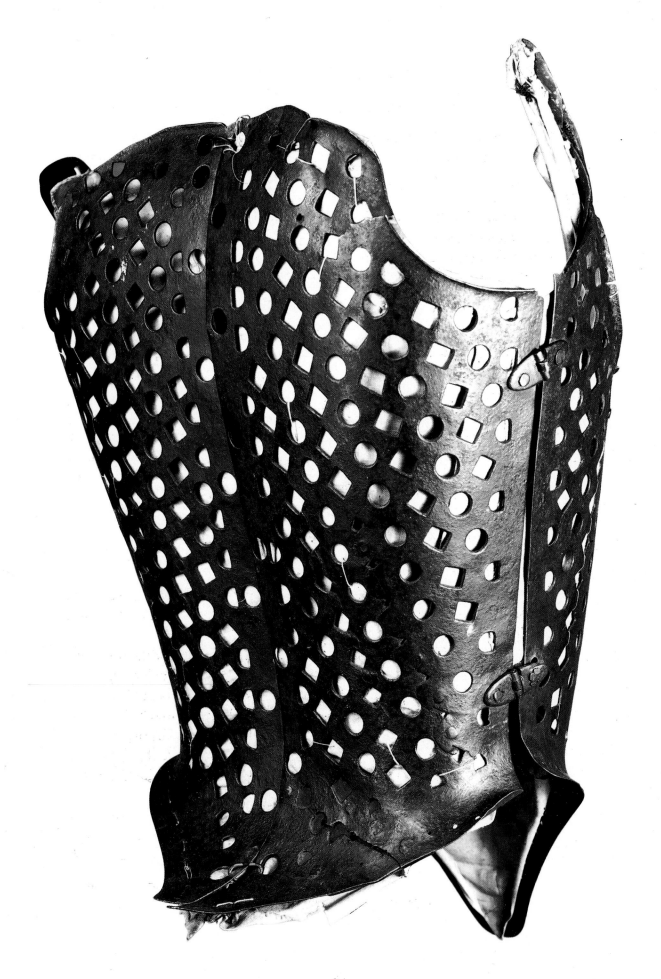

34

MAKING THE MOST OF IT

In the early sixteenth century female breasts were described as 'the devil's work'; the Pope threatened with excommunication all who 'bared their necks to excess'. Yet by the end of that same century, it was quite appropriate for Elizabethan virgins to appear in public with breasts as bare and as frank as those of the Minoan women of 2000 B.C.

Welshman Matthew Griffiths felt that this was an uncalled-for teasing display, 'If your wares bee not vendible why do you open your shoppes?' he grumbled.

Exposed bosoms in those Elizabethan times received almost as much cosmetic treatment as the face itself. Women carefully whitened their breasts with ceruse. Unfortunately, this lethal white lead paste ate viciously into the flesh, drying and corroding it and making it sore and itchy. And all the time, the toxic lead was being steadily absorbed into the bloodstream. But the appeal of ceruse was overwhelming: it made the skin look so white and radiant – at least when first applied. Later, as it etched deeper into the skin, cracks began to appear and subsequent applications had to be thicker, and yet thicker again.

At this time, too, it was commonplace for middle-aged women to paint a spidery network of blue veins on their chests to simulate the translucent skin of the very young. But the results were not always successful. As the day wore on, the whited sepulchres of their bosoms would start to itch intolerably and the marbled veins of feigned youth would invariably begin to dissolve and run.

Hiding bosoms when they are out of fashion is not so difficult as spiriting them up when fashion approves – especially for those women who are naturally flat-chested. For them, cheating is an obvious temptation. In the eighteenth century much could be done beneath the bodice to compensate for an ungenerous nature. Bust improvers known as 'waxen bosoms' or, more endearingly, 'bosom friends' became popular. These were devices made of wax or stuffed cotton. Not only were they uncomfortable to wear but with their stiff, unlifelike padding, they succeeded in fooling no one.

'Lemon' bosoms were popular in the nineteenth century and these, for the first time, introduced mobility. In 1860 a patent was taken out for the manufacture of 'an improved, inflated, undulating artificial bust'. By 1886 an enterprising gentleman from Philadelphia, Joseph Louis Wells, had introduced 'health braided wire dress forms' which he guaranteed 'do not gather dampness from perspiration . . . and can be adjusted by the wearer to any size desired'. In the same year, a French firm advertised pink rubber 'poitrines adhérentes' which were described as very successful in 'following the movements of respiration with mathematical and perfect precision'.

Even greater ingenuity in filling out a young lady's jumper was employed in Britain in the 1950s. These were the halcyon days of the sweater girl. For the under-endowed, there were high-flying brassières cunningly wired and boned to maximise every centimetre of

OPPOSITE : An iron corset from medieval Europe: up to the early sixteenth century female breasts were considered 'the devil's work' the bosom – as well as foam-rubber and oil-filled falsies, some of them remarkably realistic. There was even an inflatable bra known as 'Très Secrète'.

Magazines were full of advice. Mysterious creams, to be applied like garden fertilizers, enjoyed good sales. Vigorous exercise was recommended. Throughout Britain, determined girls filled the air with heavy breathing as they stretched, exercised their pectoral muscles and inhaled deeply to the cry – 'I must, I must, improve the bust'.

In less prosperous parts of the world more unusual attempts were made to augment the bosom. In New Guinea, girls often obtained 'a number of ants of two special kinds – their heads are pulled off, and they are rubbed on the breasts. The sharp liquid stings the skin causing slight swelling increased by dabbing with nettles.'

In some parts of southern Africa, they concentrated more on the nipple, elongating it by twisting around it strips of fibre. In Ethiopia, it was at one time reported that 'young women have their breasts so long that they reach down upon their waists, and this they take for a goodly thing and they go naked to show them for a bravery'. Again in the Kingdom of Senegal, ladies were once so keen to have 'long dugs' that they would 'have the breasts forcibly drawn out by the men who tie a rope about them for that very purpose so that they sag down to their belly'.

While in the seventeenth century publications such as J. Jeamson's *Artificiall Embellishments of Arts Best Directions* were eager to assist any ladies 'with breasts which are flaccid and hang down too low'. They were recommended to 'dissolve pitch, mix it together with oil and apply to the breasts'.

Sir Hugh Platt felt that breasts were allowable but they should be kept within limits. In his *Delightes For Ladies* he recommended that the way to 'keep breasts from growing too big' was to pickle them in vinegar:

> Put as much pounded Cummin seed into water as will suffice to make it into the consistence of a plaister, bind it when you are young somewhat, streight to the paps, with a fillet dipt in water and vinegar letting it remain three days, then take away the Cummin and apply the roots of white lillies incorporated with water, bind it likewise to the breast pretty streight and keep it on other three days . . .

Some famous women in recent times have had a great deal to say about improving chests. Princess Luciana Pignatelli is full of advice for both the 'haves' and the 'have-nots'. For those well-endowed, she is quite clear: 'Never never put your breasts in hot water, it will make them sag.'

For the benefit of others – like herself – sorely afflicted with a flat chest, she confesses all in *The Beautiful People's Beauty Book*. It was her fate to suffer the agonies of a 'protracted flat puberty'. And it was this which drove her to experiment with many things. One of her first hopeful attempts employed Niehan's cell implants, believed to be successful in developing

OPPOSITE : Jayne Mansfield, making the most of natural endowments

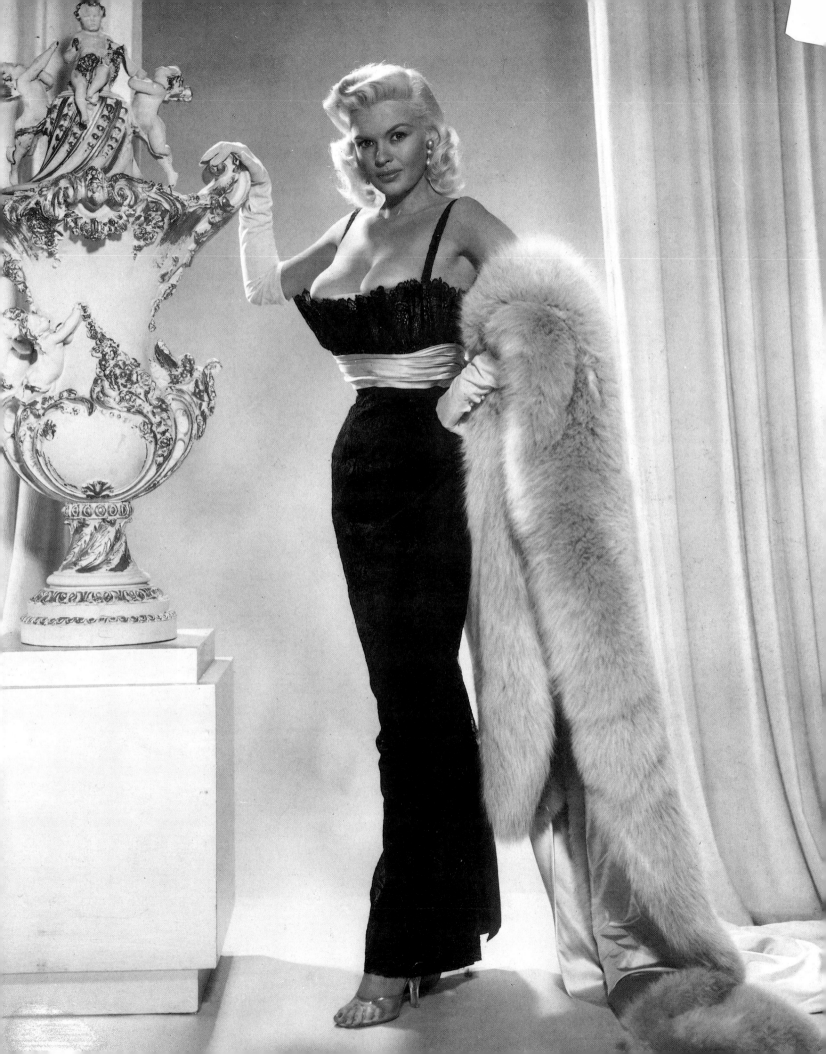

the female bosom during puberty. But they failed to work for her perhaps because – as experts patiently explained – she was well past puberty when she tried them. She then experimented with the birth-control pill and found to her great joy that she was indeed swelling, week by week. But soon, to her sorrow, all gradually subsided to her old pre-pill dimensions.

Nowadays, in Britain and America, much more drastic treatment is engaged in: more and more women seek surgery to improve their bodyline. Robert Brain, in *The Decorated Body*, is astonished at just how radical, even primitive, we are prepared to be: 'We show little reaction when we mutilate our own bodies in the interests of vanity and youthfulness . . . a woman who has learned to be ashamed of her full breasts undergoes an operation as unpleasant and as primitive as the excising of the clitoris.'

But such operations are today becoming more and more numerous. The prospect is such a tempting one. As easily as selecting a new purchase from a warehouse catalogue, a woman may order a natural-looking bosom. And – providing all goes well – she can expect to be rewarded with plenty of body and bounce. This is, of course, not always the case.

In December 1988, a 43-year-old woman was described by a judge as being 'almost obsessed with a desire to have the shape of her body altered'. Badly scarred after six breast operations, she had to have re-shaping implants removed after her left breast had hardened 'to bursting point'. She lost her case against the surgeon.

One early attempt to enlarge the bosom involved the grafting of tissue taken from the buttocks and inserted into the breast. But by the natural process of 'resorption' the new fat was always disposed of by the body and it was not long before the breast had returned to its original shape.

Another idea came from the world of 'drag'. Some female impersonators have used brassières which are really inflated balloon structures. So why not insert a balloon into the bosom itself? The idea seemed feasible, except that there was a very real possibility of air leaking into the tissues and possibly into small blood vessels which could have had fatal results. To avoid this danger, filling the balloons with fluid (salt, water and dextran) instead of air was tried. This meant inserting the deflated balloons into the breast, equipping them with small bore tubes, and pumping in the liquid. It was still necessary to avoid air leaks, especially when it was discovered that, combined with the fluid, an air leak could create a 'swish-swash' splashing sound – off-putting to the ear of an intimate in congress with the newly-inflated bosom.

In more recent years, silicone bags have proved popular for breast augmentation. One of the surgical techniques involves making a small, one-inch incision under the crease line of each breast. A silicone bag is then inserted near the rib cage to fill out the natural breast tissue. For the tiny or droopy-chested girl such a prosthesis can create firm, upward-tilting breasts simply by pushing out the skin to a more prominent, flattering shape. One

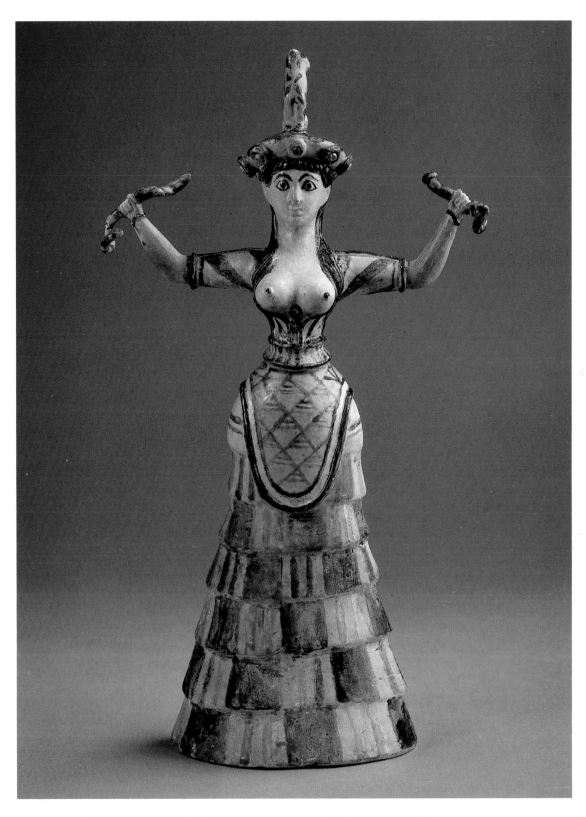

Minoan ladies of 3,000 years ago exposed their breasts in a frank, voluptuous manner complication is 'capsular contracture', the hardening of scar tissue around the implant.

But unlike silicone injections which sometimes result in an unsatisfactory 'solid' rigid bosom, the silicone gel bag – in a successful implant – has the advantage of remaining mobile and providing a lifelike 'give' on palpation. Hydrophilic gels have proved even better for the purpose. The 'Même' implant, newer and more expensive, has a foamy outer-casing, but insertion (or removal should this be needed if things go wrong) is more complicated. For this reason many surgeons choose not to use the 'Même'.

And some doctors are critical of the introduction of such materials into the breast at all, pointing out the high incidence of tumours in this area, both benign and malignant. Cosmetic surgeons, well aware of this, usually arrange to see patients who have had breast augmentation at fairly frequent intervals afterwards.

One incidental advantage of such an augmenting operation – supposing it to be a satisfactory one – is that most women can still breast-feed their babies perfectly well.

But breast-feeding is not possible following breast reduction. This operation is a major one. It is more costly, and it can go wrong. As one woman reported: 'After I came round from the operation my chest felt as if a pan of boiling oil had been poured over it. It took eleven days before the first stitches were removed and I plucked up the courage to look. I burst into tears when I saw that my left nipple was crooked and there was a lump underneath it where a stitch had been left in accidentally. This resulted in my breast becoming infected.'

There is also the risk of poor alignment following a cosmetic breast operation. A few years ago a number of Italian women emerged from operations with one breast pointing upwards and the other sideways, an asymmetry jovially labelled by the unfeeling, 'the Picasso lift'. Most women, of course, do have some slight difference in the size of their breasts, but many of the lopsided looks which have followed plastic surgery in this area have been highly distressing. Cases have occurred of nipples being positioned at different levels. Sometimes, as an added complication, hard tissue has grown around just one of the silicone bags. This, as well as being uncomfortable, has resulted in unequal-sized breasts.

Yet in spite of all the possible hazards, discomforts and expense, the number of women undergoing cosmetic breast operations is increasing each year, which is perhaps a little surprising. So many female liberationists have attempted to draw attention away from this specifically female part of the body. Yet agony aunts like Marjorie Proops continue to receive hundreds of letters from women who are worried that their busts are either too small or too big. Commercial advertising is to blame: on the one hand, Marjorie Proops writes 'the big breasted girl is universally promoted as the sexually desirable girl. [Yet] just as undue commercial breast emphasis has encouraged complexes about small breasts, so the multi-million pound slimming-aid industry has helped to create problems for the plumpish woman.'

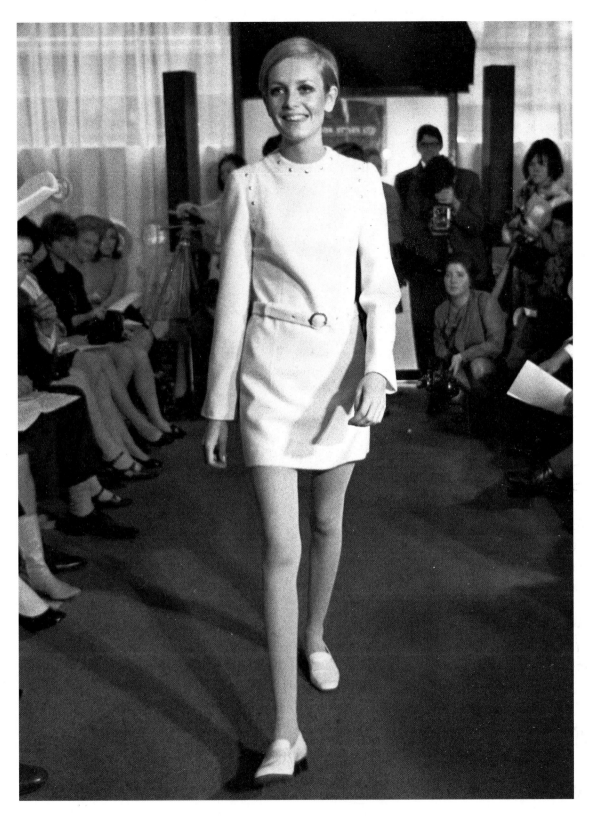

Twiggy: making the most of the least of it

Germaine Greer believed that there was no hope of consensus on bosoms because most existing stereotypes have been falsely and incorrectly generated. The 'real thing' has become obscured by the built-up, boned, heavily wired contraptions which women have so often fastened themselves into. Reality can only be restored if women refuse to wear undergarments which perpetuate the glorious masculine dream of 'pneumatic bliss'. Men admire women's breasts solely for their appearance, and just so long as they show no signs of their function. Men do not regard bosoms as a functional part of the whole woman, but rather as toys to be 'kneaded and twisted like magic putty, or munched and mouthed like lolly ices'. Once the breasts have submitted to the rigours of child-suckling – often darkening in tone and stretching – men become repelled rather than attracted by them.

But nuzzling at the breast does have its own olfactory attractions: males may not consciously be aware of its erotic odours but the glands around the nipple are, in origin, apocrine glands, and apocrine glands are the ones responsible for the special sexual scents of armpits and genitals.

No one can seriously doubt that bosoms have unmistakable sex appeal. But couturiers find that they do have one big disadvantage – they interfere with the smooth, uninterrupted flow of the dress-line. As Twiggy demonstrated in the legendary Sixties, the flat-chested girl makes an excellent clothes-horse. The French do not trouble themselves with such dilemmas: for them the chest is all-important when a girl's clothes are off, not when they are on. Naked, in the bedroom, the bosom comes into its own. Dressed and in its clothes it must take second place to the all-important line of the dress.

Yet what can be the importance of the breast today, in a world where so many women appear to be aiming at looking like men? And with such uncertain objectives. Unisex dress is chosen by equality-conscious women but frequently shows clear detail of the breasts. Women who choose to wear the collarless shirt of the stevedore often enough select it in a transparent fabric – the sort which Yves Saint Laurent used for the see-through blouse of 1968. And this, as they know full well, cannot fail to reveal the artificial nipples which many are wearing and which are often so lively and upstanding that they can only be meant to provoke.

Is the post-feminist woman now furthering her career by wearing ostensibly masculine clothes which at the same time carefully project all the old biological signals?

The Minoan women of 3,000 years ago were untroubled by any such convoluted strategies. For them there was no ambivalence about acknowledging, accepting and demonstrating their feminine endowment. Long-sleeved gowns with tight, high-waisted bodices totally without frontpieces in them, enabled these highly civilised ladies to project their busts in a frank, voluptuous display as formidable as anything on an old ship's figurehead.

3. DRESSED TO KILL

SHOWING A LEG

Cecil Beaton – possibly with tender memories of those glamorous, long-skirted, feminine dresses he created for *My Fair Lady* – spoke strongly and memorably of the mini-skirt. 'Never in the history of fashion has so little material been raised so high to reveal so much that needs to be concealed so badly.'

Not everyone, of course, would agree. For most young people the mini-skirt of the Swinging Sixties symbolised – as it still does – the new spirit of sexual freedom, and moreover, it was fun. It proclaimed the distinct change in morality that had occurred during this century. In Victorian days euphemisms like 'limbs' were required for the very word 'legs'; tables and chairs had their legs concealed by wrappings lest they should deprave the minds of observers; even chicken-legs were obliquely referred to as 'dark meat'.

When legs were finally admitted to exist beneath the quite modest knee-length skirts of the 1920s, there were still people who were outraged. Some employers refused to accept women workers in the new shorter skirts: 'half naked thighs' and legs clad in silk were provocative and they could cause the mind to wander.

The sight of men's bare legs in the knee-length khaki-shorts worn by chaps in India in the days of the Raj caused few hearts to flutter. By contrast, Bermuda shorts for day wear in the 1980s are much more arresting, though they make more demands upon their male wearers. Athletically cut – many of them in stretch Lycra and finishing just above the knee – they are causing fashionable New Yorkers to have knee-lift surgery, simply to improve their leg-look.

Even greater demands were made on men who wished to show a well-turned leg in the days of tight hose and short-skirted jackets. In the eighteenth century when 'Cavalier' high boots had gone out of fashion, men could no longer hide their leg deficiencies: those who did not possess muscular calves were forced to wear false ones if they wanted to cut a dash. But how was a man to hide this fact from a lady he wished to impress, and where was he to conceal the apparatus at the moment of truth in the boudoir? Quite a problem for the skinny-legged rococo fop. By the time he had taken his corset off and removed his two pairs of tight stockings and his calf paddings, and his wig, the lady might be having second thoughts. But no such problem for modern men whose trousers have remained, on the whole, accommodating and concealing. That is, until the arrival of jeans.

Thirty-eight million pairs of this popular garment were sold in 1976, and though in the early Eighties sales took a steep dip, by the mid-Eighties jeans were back in favour. Now,

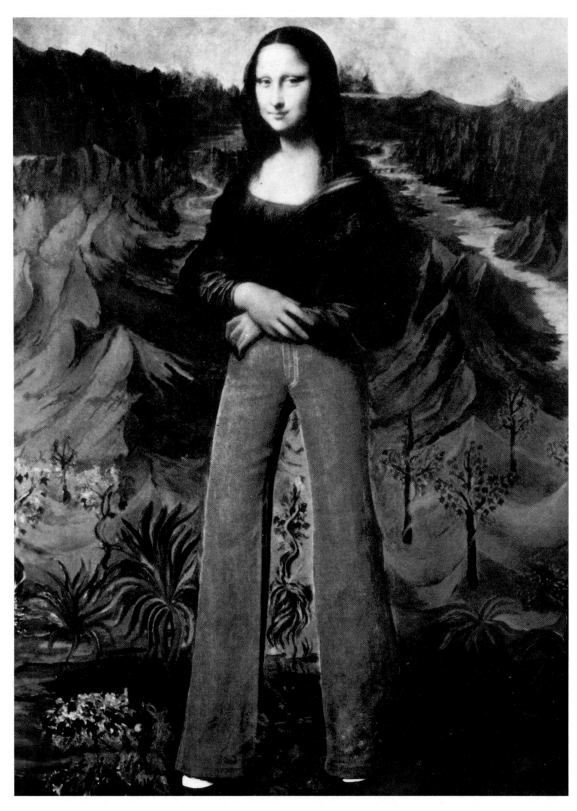

That tight-fitting jeans are as provocative as Mona Lisa's smile is the message of this 1978 ad from Foster 2 Jeans, Paris they are firmly established as a fashion classic and are clearly no longer the strictly working garment they set out to be in the mid nineteenth century.

To be impressive and truly fashionable, jeans must cling tightly to both leg and body. So perhaps it is fortunate that men's underwear no longer includes combinations and button-fronted pants, neither of which would provide a sleek foundation for today's tight jeans. Ever since Clark Gable in 1934 took off his shirt when *It Happened One Night* tough men have been buying sleeveless vests. Four years after this epochal event, the first Y-fronts appeared.

But in hot weather, snug Y-fronts under tight jeans cause perspiration which leads to chafing and infection – more succinctly – 'crotch rot'. Dr E. J. Moynaham at Guy's Hospital in London was seeing so many men with this problem in 1976 that he strongly urged the wearing of loose-fitting boxer-type pants. Other experts have seriously advocated kilts and skirts for men, which they say are a much healthier apparel, and not just because of irritating 'crotch rot'.

More serious problems are likely if men continue to overheat themselves in this sensitive area. Not for nothing does Nature arrange that male testicles are suspended outside the body in a normally cooler temperature than the 98.4°F to be found inside the body. The production of spermatazoa is best accomplished in a cool rather than a hot environment – a fact which was amply proved when men suffering from fevers and high temperatures were found to have become temporarily sterile.

Primitive tribes seem instinctively to have known about this and to have used it as a rough-and-ready form of birth control: men steep their testicles in very hot water at frequent intervals for several days before making love. As a birth control method it is chancy, and hardly to be relied on. But Bedouin tribes evidently find it useful. Constantly on the move they endeavour to orchestrate conception in their womenfolk so that birth will take place at roughly the same convenient time – when their caravanserai has rested. Their menfolk use hot compresses bandaged to the testicles. During Rommel's Desert War, some enterprising British soldiers, noting the Bedouin method, fell into the habit of setting off for a romantic assignment complete with water, primus stove, pan and bandages.

Men in the fifteenth and sixteenth centuries had few fears – on this score at least – about diminishing their sperm counts. Unlike their overheated modern descendants, these dashing gentlemen in their hot, tight hose, had the advantage of being able to cool off in their cod-pieces.

The hemline for men in the 1340s was on the knee but by the 1360s – to the consternation of many – it had risen to mid-thigh. The Parson in Chaucer's *Canterbury Tales* clearly disapproved: 'Alas! Some of them show the very boss of the penis and the horrible pushed out testicles that look like the malady of hernia in the wrapping of their hose.'

By the mid-fifteenth century jackets had crept up so short and stockings were so tight, they left little to the imagination. For modesty's sake some sort of accommodation for a man's genitals had to be adopted. Protective cod-pieces had already been worn by warrior knights – now they were re-introduced for fashionable cover-up purposes. But by the time fashion had finished with them, they were anything but a cover-up. They grew more and more commodious, and were often so splendidly bejewelled that they could hardly fail to direct attention to that which they were supposed to be ignoring. Occasionally, they were used to house a few treasures, sometimes even a sweetmeat snack or two. To excite the imagination further they were quite unnecessarily padded and suggestively stiffened. Nowadays, to add lustre – and bulk – to their presentation a number of male pop-stars employ judicious padding. Others – in the manner of a heavy-bosomed lady heaving herself into her bra – achieve a revealing high-line crotch by uncomfortably uplifting themselves inside skin-tight trousers.

Women have not had quite the same problems though nylon tights have often enough been responsible for foot deformities caused by constricted toes. And these days, jeans are beginning to generate medical problems. To acquire a body-line fit, many women are prepared to climb into them (often having to lie down to get them on at all) and then lie in a shallow bath of water so that the jeans will shrink revealingly to the body. Hardly a healthy prescription for the capillaries and arteries.

Women are complaining of upper-leg skin problems caused by chafe. Dermatologists are seeing sufferers from a new kind of vanity-thrush, women plagued by itching skin, who only reluctantly are being persuaded to loosen their jeans to get rid of their rash.

In August 1985 a Cornish woman on holiday collapsed on a Scottish moor. Police investigating discovered that in the heavy rain, her body-tight jeans had tightened so much they had cut off the blood supply to her legs.

OPPOSITE : Originally introduced for cover-up purposes, cod-pieces became unnecessarily padded and suggestively stiffened. The illustration shows Prince Don Carlos of Spain (1545–1568)

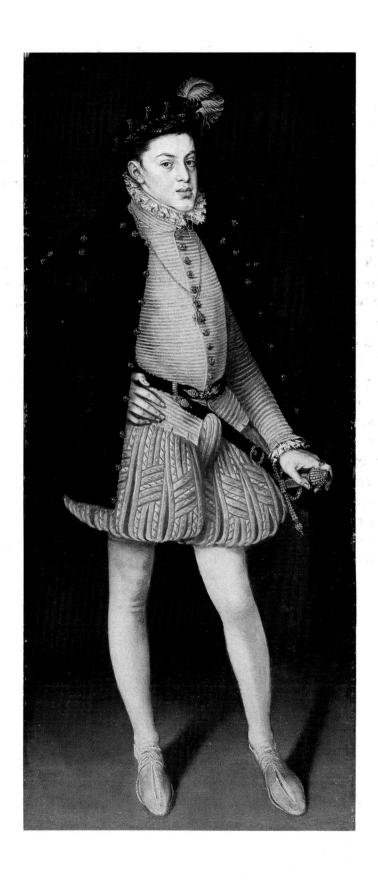

BODY BONDAGE

In earlier times too, women have had their share of collapsing. The sight of a fragile-looking lady in grave difficulties with a heaving bosom might have caused sympathetic observers in the nineteenth century to assume that she was in the grip of some great emotion. She was much more likely, however, to be experiencing difficulty in breathing. Her tightly-laced corset was probably pressing upwards into her lungs so hard and downwards into her abdomen so fiercely that normal breathing was impossible. An X-ray photograph would amost certainly have revealed a damaged liver as well as a displaced rib or two. But in the nineteenth century some sort of mid-riff constriction was necessary because fashion required a small waist. And few women would have argued with that.

One contemporary journal put it: 'If the various organs are prevented from taking a certain form or direction they will accommodate themselves to anything with perfect ease.'

Unfortunately, this is not the view of modern medical science. It is now abundantly clear that addiction in the past to tiny, emaciated waists has caused all kinds of mutilation, injury to internal organs, chest diseases, sometimes death. And one thing on which all are now agreed is that the major culprit was that supremo of strait-jackets, the corset. For of all the many aids to stylish beauty the corset must surely have been fashion's most sinister henchman. Yet the corset reigned with rod of iron, steel, wood and whalebone for six hundred tyrannical years – a torturing contrivance which made women faint, gasp with pain, fall over and quite literally hold their breath.

But women have always shown themselves willing to punish their bodies to achieve a slender-mid-riff look. In ancient Greece mothers bound their babies to keep them thin and to increase their height. They made no allowance for any movement of the arms until the child was six months old. Even Plato – wise in so many other things – said that this should continue until the child was two years old. Some vain mothers carried on winding bands of wool or linen around the torsos of their infant daughters well beyond babyhood, in the hope that the girls would grow up tall and slender.

In Chaucer's time a tiny waist came to be a sign of great gentility. To achieve it, ladies used a stiffened , linen underbodice made from a sandwich of two layers of fabric with paste in the middle. Christened the 'cotte' (from the French côte) this bone-pressing sandwich was the earliest form of corset.

At one stage, small boards – about two inches wide – were introduced into the close-fitting fabric bodices, with strings attached for tighter lacing. To encourage an even narrower V-shaped frontage, women also took to placing lead plates on their breasts. Many began to find they could not nurse their babies. Others fainted when the apparatus was removed and found it safer to continue wearing their lead companions, even in bed.

Not content with this masochistic orgy, women weighted themselves down with cumbersome dresses made from heavy and elaborate fabrics. This extra luxury involved a further problem: to do the heavy fabrics justice and allow them to hang gracefully, some sort of framework supported at the waist was needed. At first cages, unwieldy and heavy, were tried. Until suddenly from Spain came a much more ingenious solution. It was called the farthingale and in one form or another, it remained popular for three hundred years.

The early farthingales usually began with a cone or bell-shaped framework at the waist. Then came several petticoats and a padded 'stomacher'. The fashionable lady added to this padded shoulders and arms, and even a couple of pairs of stockings or socks. Fully dressed, she was weighed down beyond all reason. Queen Elizabeth I's doubtful temper in later years is sometimes attributed to the enormous weight of ceremonial clothes she was obliged to drag around with her.

With so much attire to attend to it is hardly surprising that the sixteenth-century lady was always fidgety, forever looking about her to see how all her bits and pieces were faring. And there was another, more urgent cause for her generally unsettled state – within her apparel there were uninvited but distinctly lively guests. Her costume with so much padding and bulk of cloth provided a perfect paradise for lice and fleas.

Yet replete with livestock, these women made their appearance at fêtes, ballets and masquerades, undaunted, magnificently attired and often, so it was said 'so laden with precious stones that they could not move about'.

The corset underlying all this finery could hardly be described as a help to mobility either. For by this time it had become 'a hard and solid mould into which the wearer had to be compressed there to remain and suffer, in spite of the splinters of wood that penetrated the flesh, took the skin off the waist and made the ribs ride up one over the other'.

'Women strive all that they possibly can by straight-lacing themselves to attain unto a wand-like smallness of waiste, never thinking themselves fine enough until they can span their waiste,' wrote the playwright, John Bulwer, in 1650, 'and to that end by strong compulsion shut up their waistes in a whalebone prison in little ease; they open a door to consumption and a withering rottenness'.

The philosopher John Locke took up the same theme forty years later: 'Narrow breasts, short and stinking breath, ill lungs and crookedness are the natural and almost constant effects of hard bodice and clothes that pinch.'

But women ignored their many critics. At the time they were far too preoccupied with the requirements of a new type of skirt called the 'panier'. Width, rather than circumference, was the basis of its style. To be truly in the fashion petticoat hoops were recklessly extended more and more to right and to left until – throwing all caution to the winds and regardless of accommodation problems – ladies blossomed and took off in skirts of anything up to two yards wide. In France, according to one observer: 'Everyone laughed. Here were several ladies to be accommodated in a coach which could hold only one with her balloon skirt. Everything was too small; the streets were too narrow, the salon doors

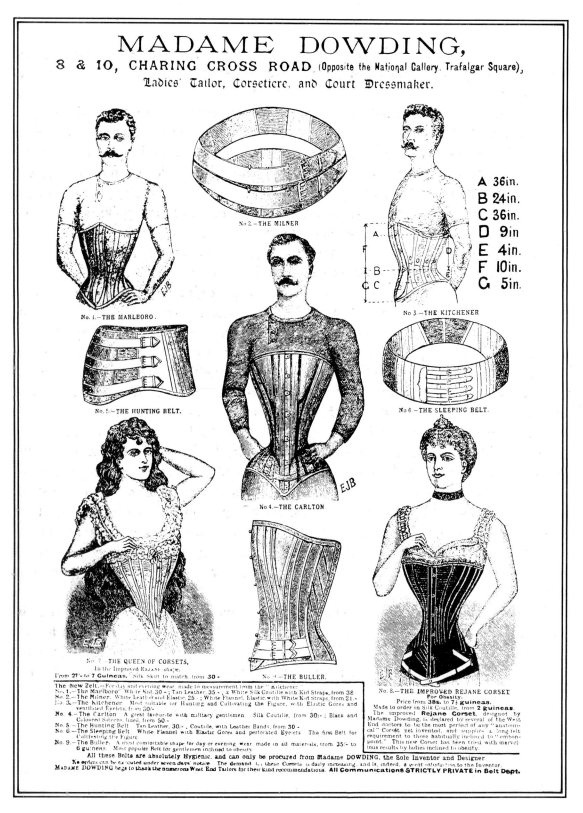

MADAME DOWDING,

8 & 10, CHARING CROSS ROAD (Opposite the National Gallery, Trafalgar Square),
Ladies' Tailor, Corsetiere, and Court Dressmaker.

No 2.—THE MILNER

A 36in.
B 24in.
C 36in.
D 9in.
E 4in.
F 10in.
G 5in.

No. 1.—THE MARLBORO.

No. 3.—THE KITCHENER

No. 5.—THE HUNTING BELT.

No. 6.—THE SLEEPING BELT.

No. 4.—THE CARLTON

No. 7.—THE QUEEN OF CORSETS,
In the Improved Rejane shape.
From 21/- to 7 Guineas. Silk Skirt to match, from 30/-

No. 9.—THE BULLER.

No. 8.—THE IMPROVED REJANE CORSET
For Obesity.
Price from 38s. to 7½ guineas.
Made to order in Silk Coutille, from 2 guineas.
The improved **Rejane Corset**, designed by Madame Dowding, is declared by several of the West End doctors to be the most perfect of any "anatomical" Corset yet invented, and supplies a long felt requirement to those habitually inclined to "embonpoint." This new Corset has been tried with marvellous results by ladies inclined to obesity.

The New Zelt.—For day and evening wear, made to measurement from the "Kitchener"
No. 1.—The Marlboro' White Kid, 30/-; Tan Leather, 35/-; x White Silk Coutille with Kid Straps, from 38/-
No. 2.—The Milner. White Leather and Elastic, 25/-; White Flannel, Elastic with White Kid Straps, from 21/-
No. 3.—The Kitchener. Most suitable for Hunting and Cultivating the Figure, with Elastic Gores and ventilated Eyelets, from 30/-
No. 4.—The Carlton. A great favourite with military gentlemen. Silk Coutille, from 30/-; Black and Coloured Sateens lined, from 50/-
No. 5.—The Hunting Belt. Tan Leather, 30/-; Coutille, with Leather Bands, from 30/-
No. 6.—The Sleeping Belt. White Flannel with Elastic Gores and perforated Eyelets. The first Belt for Cultivating the Figure
No. 9.—The Buller. A most comfortable shape for day or evening wear, made in all materials, from 35/- to 6 guineas. Most popular Belt for gentlemen inclined to obesity.

All these Belts are absolutely Hygienic, and can only be procured from Madame DOWDING, the Sole Inventor and Designer
No orders can be executed under seven days' notice. The demand for these Corsets is daily increasing, and is, indeed, a great satisfaction to the Inventor.
MADAME DOWDING begs to thank the numerous West End Tailors for their kind recommendations. All Communications STRICTLY PRIVATE in Belt Dept.

In Edwardian times, men were as committed as women to hour-glass figures, often risking internal damage to organs had to be widened to allow the ladies to pass in, just as it became necessary afterwards to make the doors higher at the top so that the gigantic headdresses of later days might enter without a hitch.'

The men were full of grumbles. From looking as though they had 'bums like barrels' ladies now walked 'as if they were in a go-cart'. But, when women started to wear flimsier materials over their hoops instead, these lightweight fabrics were often revealingly blown about – even turned inside-out – by the wind. Gentlemen, suddenly full of concern and interest, rushed to their aid. Mrs Haywood, in *The Female Spectator* of 1744, felt moved to report with ingenuous wonder: 'What manner some ladies come into public assemblies – they do not walk but straddle and sometimes run with a kind of frisk and jump, throw their enormous hoops almost in the face of those who pass them. The men of these times', she went on, 'are strangely happy'. Perhaps even 'cock-a-hoop'?

A few changes did come towards the end of the eighteenth century when, quite suddenly, with one of those sudden convulsions which happen so often in fashion, high-waisted muslin gowns became all-at-once popular. Very light and clinging to the figure, these revealing frocks were frequently worn with very little beneath them. Sometimes, for piquancy and variety, women deliberately dampened their cotton and muslin dresses to make them cling appealingly to the body – in spite of the fact that everyone knew they were in danger of going down with chills or pneumonia.

In Napoleon's heyday, a 13-inch waist was considered to be just about ideal. It was not unusual, said one account of 1810, 'to see a mother lay her daughter down upon the carpet, placing her foot on her back, and break half a dozen laces in tightening her stays'.

An irate tradesman of 1828 complained: 'My daughters are living instances of the baleful consequences of the dreadful fashion of squeezing the waist until the body resembles that of an ant. They are unable to stand, sit or walk as women used to do. My daughter Margaret made the experiment the other day: her stays gave way with a tremendous explosion and down she fell upon the ground. I thought she had snapped in two.'

The crinoline made its dramatic entrance in the years of the new young Queen Victoria. Its enormous volume was supported by bulky petticoats but it was also provided with many ingenious devices for holding it out. Air-filled tubes were tried, gathered together in the form of a huge bell. In May 1856, a patent was taken out for an inflatable garment which could be conveniently deflated when its owner wished to sit down. However, the heavy bellows which needed carrying around for pumping up the dress when the lady wished to – as it were – come up for air, were distinctly inconvenient. And the inevitable noises disconcerting.

In the drawing-room crinolines were killers. They were notorious for touching the open firegrate without the wearer's knowledge. With such highly inflammable materials, there was immediately an inferno and little could be done – the bulky framework made it impossible to roll the victim in anything like a blanket or a rug.

But the crinolines grew ever more vast and the tightly laced corsets underpinning them continued to be worn. And now informed fears were being expressed as to their bad effects on the internal organs of women. Attention was drawn to the work of the Prussian anatomist Samuel Thomas von Sömmering who had written a paper in 1788 outlining the dangerous consequences of corsets. He had contrasted the skeleton of the Medici Venus with the skeleton of a tightly-laced woman; the difference was remarkable. Since that time, the 'tight-girdle syndrome' has become recognised in medicine as 'Sömmering's Syndrome'.

One very interesting suggestion has been made by David Kunzle. Did these women cling to their corsets as a libertarian reprieve from constant child-bearing? That the Victorian corset did endanger women's child-bearing ability is not in doubt. *The Lancet* of 1868 was quite clear: 'The mischief produced by such a practice [of wearing stays] can hardly be over-estimated. It tends gradually to displace all the most important organs of the body while by compressing them it must, from the first, interfere with their functions.' In 1874, a book by a certain 'Luke Limner' (John Leighton) attributed no fewer than 97 diseases to the wearing of tight stays.

In the end, it was women themselves who took effective action. Lady Harberton founded the Rational Dress Society in 1881, to 'promote the cause of health, comfort, and sense in dress'. The Society's publication, *The Gazette*, campaigned vigorously against tight-lacing, crinolines and high heels, and specified a maximum of no more than seven pounds in weight for underwear, a weight which today would be judged far too heavy.

But just as Chinese women tottered and fell when they cast off their foot bindings (see Ch. 9), so corseted women discovered just how much they also had become dependent on their shackles. The dense material and tight-lacing of the corset – plus the uncomfortable deportment boards which many Victorian women wore strapped to their backs – had undoubtedly provided a measure of support, albeit painful. A vicious circle had been created. Women felt weakened and lost without their stays.

It was only when Dr Jaeger invented the 'sanitary woollen spring corset' that ladies were able at last to enjoy 'all the advantages of girded loins without the disadvantages'. Made of undyed sheep's wool in white and grey and camel hair, with steels buttoned at the upper end so that they could be removed for cleaning, the Jaeger corset was described as 'flexible, elastic, durable, with watchspring steels'. And women, everywhere, welcomed it.

But then, in 1911, a particularly tight, calf-length skirt appeared. This 'hobble skirt' was the inspiration of Paul Poiret who piously declared that he had 'waged war on the corset to give free play to the abdomen but', he added triumphantly, 'I shackled the legs.' Women complained they could no longer get into their carriages. Yet their complaints seemed only to increase the popularity of this perverse fashion.

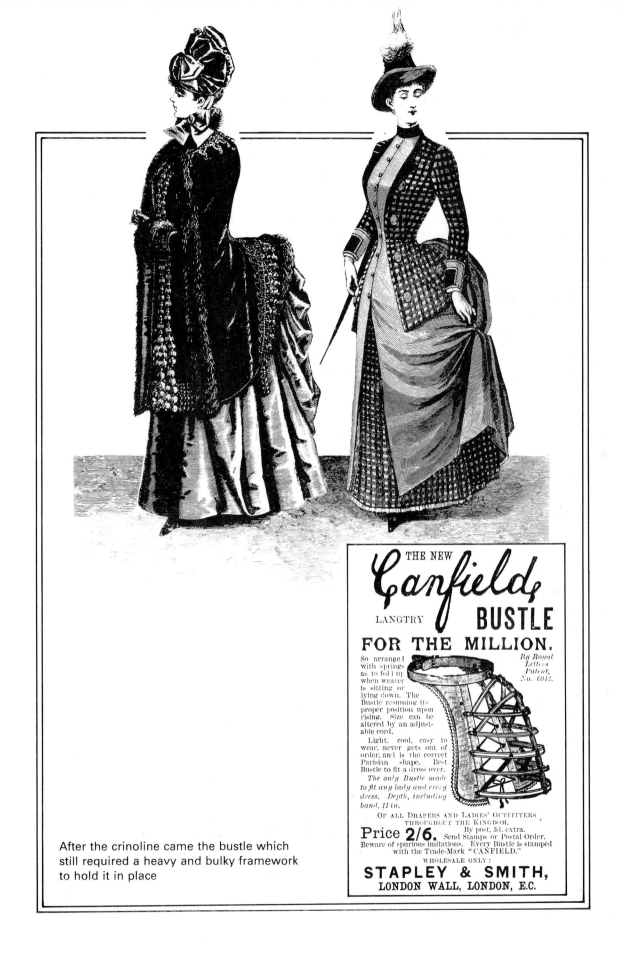

After the crinoline came the bustle which still required a heavy and bulky framework to hold it in place

By the late 1950s the female shape had gone through several changes from the bosomless flapper back to large bosoms and tiny waists. Gina Lollobrigida's much publicised 19-inch waist became an important part of her image. Dior – in the immediate post-war period – required a 17-inch waist from his models. This, he declared, was something to be attained 'even if the wearer faints'. The journal *Le Corset de France*, in 1949, was more reasonably prepared to settle for 20 inches.

In the 1950s, couturiers' models frequently used boned bras and abbreviated corsets. Sometimes the dresses themselves were boned. Penelope Portrait, top model of these times, described one monstrosity which she had to wear as 'The Iron Maiden'. Jacques Fath is rumoured to have mercilessly starved his mannequins in addition to imprisoning them in tight corsets. They were reported as gasping for air as dressers prepared them for their entrances. But in Japan, women have suffered this for generations. The broad sash – or obi – of the traditional kimono is bound so tightly around the wearer that Japanese ladies often beg to be rescued from it.

Now towards the end of the 1980s, there is much more freedom of choice particularly in the West. An 'anything goes' spirit has begun to offer women the opportunity to express themselves; conventions have been relaxed. Troublesome accessories too have declined. Hats are no longer a 'must' even for formal events – trousers are acceptable for all but the most formal occasions. Skirts can be long or short, dresses close or loose-fitting.

A corset around the neck seems improbable at first glance. But in the interests of beauty Burmese ladies have willingly submitted to having their necks encased in a succession of brass rings. They start with five rings when they are children and work up to anything between twenty-two and twenty-four. In the process their necks are elongated and the vertebrae so pulled apart and the clavicle cramped downwards to form part of the body, that a neck has been known to measure 15¾ inches. Stripped of their rings these 'giraffe-necked' women would no longer be able to support the weight of their head and would, in all probability, die.

The Elizabethans had been pleased to draw attention to their necks by surrounding them with ruffs. The bigger the ruff the more aristocratic the woman, so ruffs soared to such a height and width that they too needed supporting. The timely introduction of starch in 1564 by a Dutch woman, Madame Dingham Vander Plasse, was a great help. But after a time, the stiffly-starched moat around the chin became so vast and so impregnable, ladies found it difficult to eat. Catherine de Medicis had to have special, long-handled cutlery made.

This notion of indicating aristocratic origins through dress and bodily features is common enough. Large ruffs, small waists, tiny feet, elaborate hairstyles, smooth complexions and grossly impractical fingernails have all been used to hint at a high-born, leisurely lifestyle.

OPPOSITE : Burmese women have been known to stretch their necks to a length of 15¾ inches. Without their rings, their necks would no longer be able to support their heads

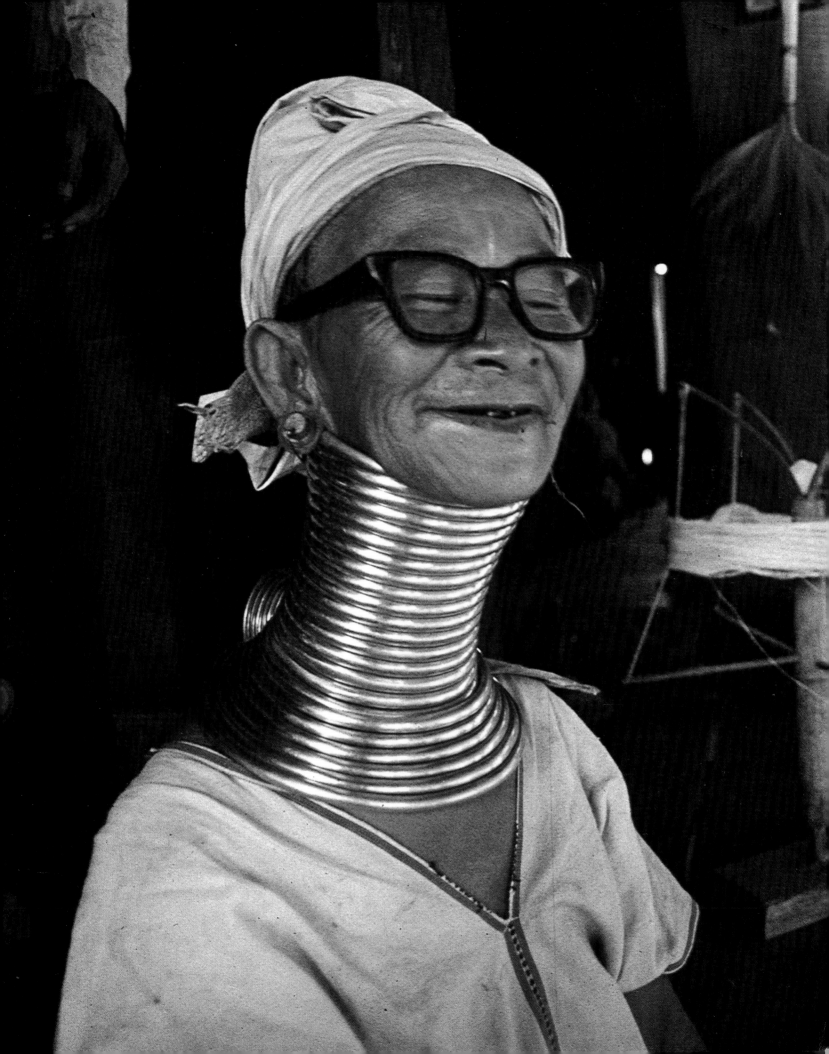

In ancient China, for reasons of prestige, both men and women grew their nails long and painted them gold. Then they spent tedious hours resting them on cushions. Later on, preferring to use their hands more, but still wishing to indicate their nobility, they compromised and confined the habit to their little fingers only. In some Mediterranean countries, young men still grow one little fingernail long, to signal that they are not rough workers. But the record for ultimate length must go to the Indian, Shrindhar Cillal of Poona, who has given thirty years of devoted care to the growing of his left-hand fingernails. Taken together his nails were found to measure almost 116 inches with his thumb nail alone measuring 29½ inches. Mr Cillal's left hand enjoys a complete life of leisure, his right one deals with all day-to-day matters.

SKIN-PICS

For many naked peoples, decorating the body offers opportunities for aesthetic satisfaction as well as having deep symbolic significance. For any dark-skinned peoples, especially, the intricate patterns created by painful incising of the flesh and raising of scars is far more effective than tattooing.

The ancient Greeks and Romans lavished a great deal of time and care on their bodily skin. They admired the naked body but found it more beautiful when it was honed and depilated to the smoothness of statuary. And this was often most painfully undertaken – either by plucking, or rubbing with pumice-stone, or even singeing.

The Japanese have different ideas. In their opinion there is nothing glorious or beautiful about a nude. The anthropologist Robert Brain tells of the Japanese view: 'Unfortunately horrible is the sight of the naked body. It really does not have the slightest charm.'

Perhaps this lack of appreciation of the bare body accounts for the fact that it is rarely depicted in erotic drawings. For the Japanese, it is not the naked body which stimulates sexual arousal; for them the true excitement is roused by a body which is richly tattooed. Which is no doubt why men have their genitals tattooed, sometimes so as to represent a plum or an aubergine. This, however, can be very demanding: since the design only comes into its own when the penis is erect, periods of long-sustained tumescence are required while the practitioner is at work. Women prostitutes in Japan sometimes engage in artful tattooing too, using sensuous snake images on the upper thighs, clearly intended to convey an erotic message.

For a Maori chief his intricately-worked facial tattoo was of fundamental importance – it was his signature. To 'sign' a document – perhaps to authorise a land sale – he would draw his own personal 'moko' tattoo. And these complex designs were so prized that on the field of battle the head of a dead warrior would often be cut off and carefully preserved; his fallen friend, with an undecorated face, was ignored.

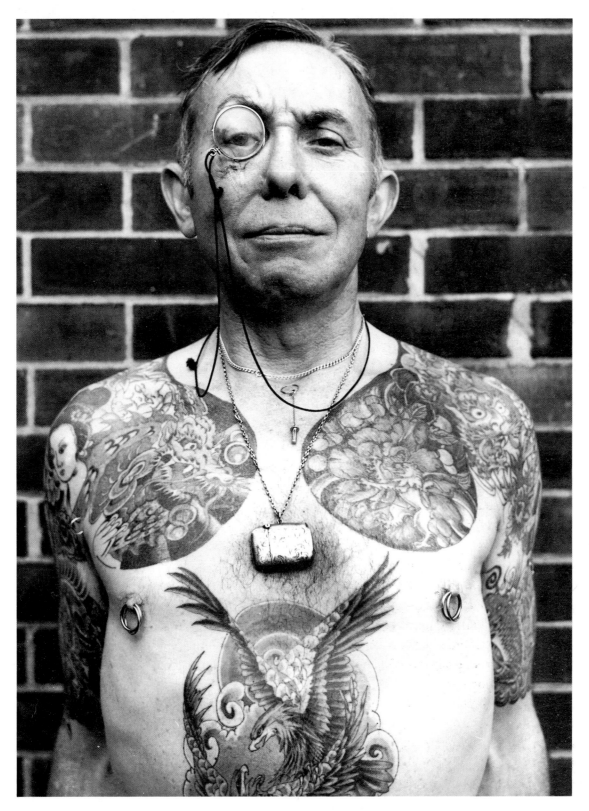

The tattoos of this British civil servant have cost him 137 hours of pain. His body is almost totally covered with bizarre designs

In New Guinea, tattoos mark a young girl's progress towards womanhood. As a child, her hands and arms are tattooed and later – when she is considered ready for marriage – her buttocks and face. Trobriand girls of Melanesia were often tattooed round the vagina at the menarche.

Egyptian mummies dating from 2000 B.C. have been discovered, decorated by tattooing. And in medieval Britain, some tattooing was practised, though the church was strongly against it. Nonetheless, in 1066, the body of Harold at Hastings was found to have 'Edith' inscribed over the heart.

But it was Captain Cook, after one of his voyages to Tahiti in 1769, who re-introduced tattooing to the West. Accompanied by the spectacular 'Great Omai', a dramatically decorated Polynesian, he made a tour of the finest drawing-rooms in London, and created a new interest in the art. By the time the celebrated and highly-skilled George Burchett had set up practice in London, the British aristocracy were ready to try it for themselves. Burchett had been taught his skills in Japan, and soon had the distinction of working on the Duke of York (the future King George V), Tsar Nicholas of Russia, and others, as well as Lady Randolph Churchill who wished to celebrate the coronation of Edward VII.

Nowadays, young people all over Europe rejoice in the habit and have their faces and bodies tattooed with pretty pictures, affirmations of romantic love, allegiance to favourite pop-stars and in the spirit of the age, defiant aggressive slogans.

A series of International Tattoo Conventions was launched in the Seventies which has given opportunities for the dedicated to exchange ideas. And not only the young are involved. In 1988, a top civil servant confessed that he likes the shock he creates by wearing an open-necked shirt to give a glimpse of his tattoos – especially when he happens to be wearing his monocle. His body, no longer young, is almost totally covered with bizarre designs which have cost him £2,000 and 137 hours of pain.

The pain of tattooing is inescapable. And there are always dangers. Lead, cadmium and mercury dyes were regularly employed as late as the 1890s. The pigments used by some so-called 'backward' societies were much less likely to cause skin problems, though their 'surgical implements' – pieces of bone or shark's teeth – were hardly aseptic and caused unbelievable pain. Opium was often used to relieve the sufferer.

In the past few years, fear of the AIDS virus has brought a decline in the number of enthusiasts. It is so difficult to be convinced that a needle is new or correctly sterilised and some customers no longer feel secure. Staff at AIDS helplines warn of the dangers of infection but there are still customers who remain undaunted. As one young man said as he was having a large eagle and skull inscribed on his leg: 'Some people collect Van Goghs or Rembrandts. I collect tattoos.'

The great problem with all tattoos is how to get rid of them. Names of old sweethearts can, it is true, be overprinted, some more successfully than others. A lover dedicating

OPPOSITE: The work of leading London tattooist, Dennis Cockell

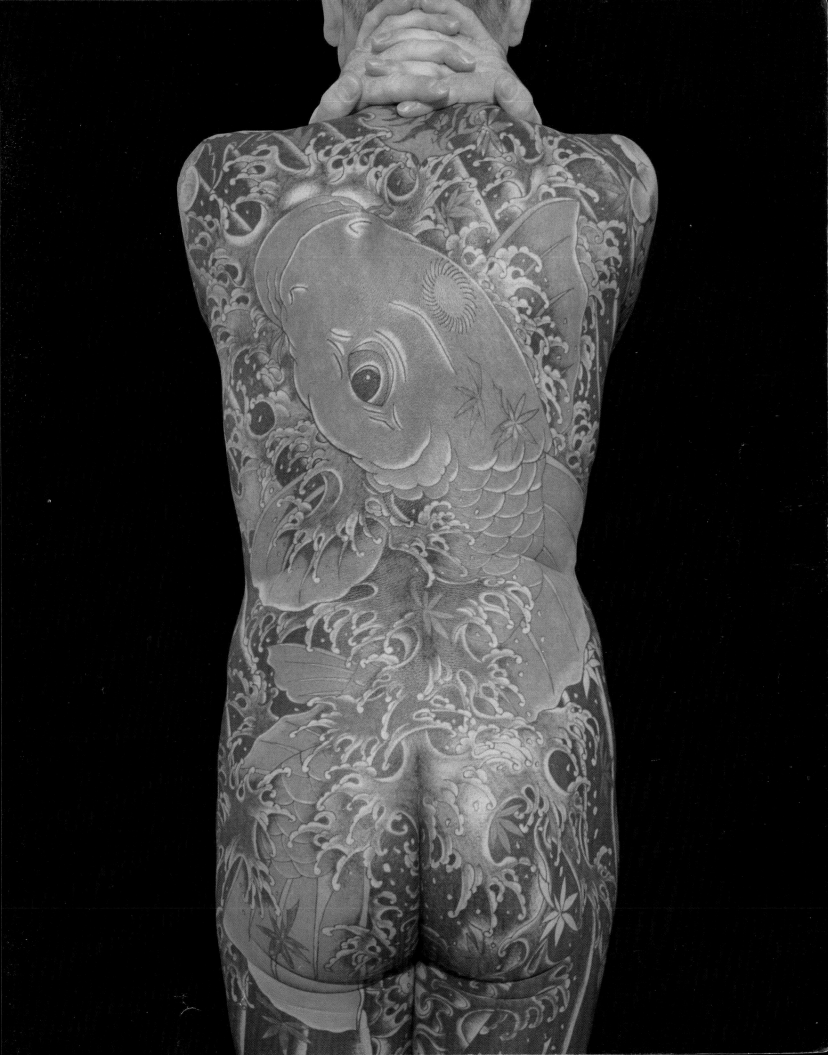

himself to Annie might well – if he should tire of her – look around for an Alice, a more convenient replacement than say Rosemary (for remembrance?) though Rosemary would be highly convenient after Mary!

The technique that has to be used is the rotating wire brush method known as dermabrasion – which involves penetration of the skin sufficiently to reach the deeper layers which pigments have penetrated. This is hardly a comfortable process and frequently produces secondary scarring. One method, introduced by Clabaughin, in 1968 in the United States, is capable of removing frozen skin segments. If followed by gentian violet dressings which give a crust to the wound, it is sometimes successful. But removing the pigment by stimulating the body's own cell scavengers – which is what is believed to happen – is an interference not to everyone's liking.

Tattoos – those 'pigments of the imagination' as photographer Chris Wroblewski has described them – are not without their problems. Where beauty is literally skin deep, a change of mind, or heart, can bring painful penalties.

A FOURTH DIMENSION – SMELL

The ancient Greeks used special scents for each part of the body: marjoram for the hair, apple-juice for the hands. At great dinners, Athenian youths were employed to saturate doves with all kinds of aromatic oils. At a suitable moment, the birds were set free to flutter over the banqueting table, filling the air with the perfumed flapping of clipped wings.

The Romans employed human scent sprays – slaves who filled their mouths with sweet-smelling waters which they blew over the heads of mistresses and guests. The Emperor Nero – more technically inclined – fitted sprays to the painted ceilings of his banqueting hall to envelop Poppaea and her guests in gentle mists of perfume.

Elizabethan men and women were not so fortunate. Their garments were often so elaborate they were unwashable, sanitary arrangements were rudimentary and baths virtually unknown. But they made the best of things by swinging scented pomanders and spent their time chewing vigorously on cloves to mask odours from foul teeth.

Nowadays, however squeaky clean we feel we are, we still seek artificial fragrances; 'body odour' has such a terrifying ring about it. The armpits, the pubic zone, the breath, the hair, are all hotbeds of psychological concern and anxiety. So we pit our wits against nature with soaps, lotions – even chlorophyll drugs – to remove every last trace of our shameful exudations. But perspiration is an essential natural mechanism and its prevention by chemicals can cause blockage and possibly rupture of the sweat ducts. Use of perspiration inhibitors over large areas of the body, particularly in hot climates is especially undesirable. Yet in the UK alone sales of deodorants and anti-perspirants now exceed £50 million a year. The availability of these in aerosol form has encountered much opposition

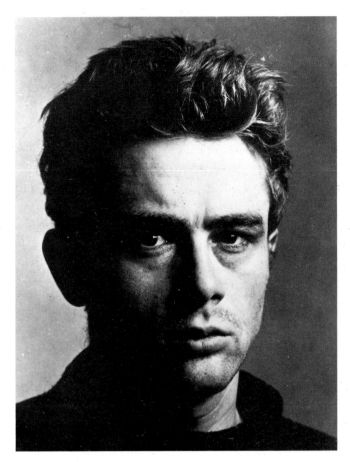

James Dean: Rebel without a Bath

from environmentalists fearful of their effects on the earth's ozone layer. Fortunately there are alternatives.

Advertisers unremittingly remind us of our aromas, even the most intimate. Yet chemical interference can have unpleasant consequences. One vulval deodorant contains chlorhexidine hydrochloride which can cause very unpleasant reactions in some female users.

The trouble with most of our secretions, especially those from the armpits and pubic areas, is that they are mixed with perspiration which can all too easily become offensive by the action of bacteria which generate acrid-smelling butyric acid when allowed to remain any time on skin and clothing. Not that everyone finds this undesirable. Some celebrated people – for one reason or another – have been reluctant to part with their own special smells. James Dean, cult star of the 1950's *Rebel Without a Cause* never took a bath. Boxer Alan Minter believed in remaining unwashed for a week to 'psych' his opponents – no-one wanted to stay long in clinches. Frenchman Joey Girondelle used a similar strategy; he

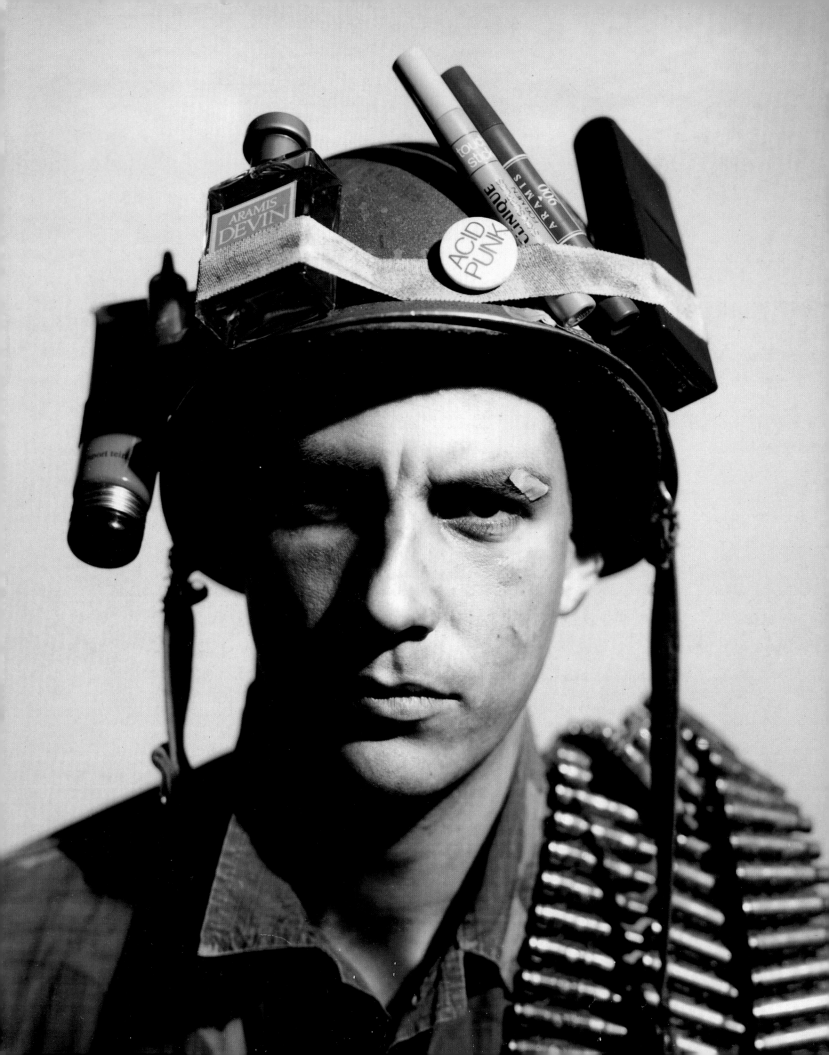

munched a clove of garlic before stepping into the ring. And Marilyn Monroe was renowned among her close associates for letting Nature speak for herself.

Perhaps she knew what she was doing: some very interesting substances are produced by the apocrine glands. These complex chemicals – the pheromones – have been evolved by Nature to bring us together and make us physically attractive to one another. We do not even need to be aware of them, yet we can quite unconsciously be stirred by them. Throughout the animal kingdom they are powerful agents in transmitting important messages. A millionth of a millionth of a gram is all that is needed to trigger a response and to bring about mating behaviour. Moths, for example, can be attracted from a mile away.

Human smells are more complicated. Male pheromones have even been shown, in certain circumstances, to influence female menstrual cycles.

The essential oils – musks and perfumes originally used simply to mask body odours – are now marketed on their sex-appeal. They promise glamour, acceptance, reward. A swooning female demonstrates the ecstasy of giving herself up to the exotic pleasures of the perfume 'Opium'. The House of Worth have pursued a discreet, ongoing storyline in their marketing. 'Je Reviens' they promised first. 'Vers toi' they said next. And when else would 'I Return', 'Towards You', save (as in their third in the series) . . . 'Dans La Nuit'?

Men too are being enticed into anointing themselves. By the 1980s the male market for fragrances with masculine titles like 'Chaps', 'Macho', 'Brut', had risen to £70 million in the UK and in America nearly 1,000 million dollars.

The name, of course, is crucial: for the more diffident gentleman who has not yet dared a seductive dab behind the ear, 'bath products' may seem more acceptable. Radox offer a healthy-sounding 'Herbal Bath'. Badedas suggest mysteriously that 'Things happen after a Badedas Bath'. Perhaps they do; both products contain horse-chestnut which has – as the Marquis de Sade noted in one of his more robust stories – a peculiarly insistent aroma. Horse-chestnut in flower is semen-like in smell.

Perfume technicians are almost always men. In the trade they are known to have keener noses than women. As well as being sensitive to the subtle differences in the essential oils from crushed flower petals, they are experienced in the qualities of animal products – secretions of civet cats, and musk deer and ambergris from the sperm whale. Yet in this area, women do have one very special talent: they are a thousand times more sensitive to detecting musk-like smells than are men. With ovaries removed this talent in women disappears. But administration of the sex hormone oestrogen brings it back – clear evidence once again of the subtle interrelationships of sex and smell.

O P P O S I T E : Male cosmetics are now a huge industry and likely to increase

4. THE FACE:
CHANGING THE COLOUR

More than 1,500 million pounds are spent each year on beauty products in the West – another fifty million pounds a year simply to advertise them. And the figures keep on climbing. It is difficult to escape the conclusion that there exists an uncontrollable urge to decorate ourselves, above all to colour ourselves, whatever the risks, the dangers, the expense.

Western society is not alone in this of course. Women and men right across the world have been engaged in this strange love affair with paints and potions for quite literally thousands of years. In ancient Egypt every Pharaoh made sure that his tomb was supplied with seven different pots of salve and two pots of rouge for the time when his ghost would return to his body; at neolithic burials, containers of red ochre were placed near corpses to provide colour for the afterlife.

And it is always the face which stimulates the greatest desire to experiment. On to this – our most visible target for improvement – we have heaped creams, lotions, lead paint, brimstone, mercury, blood, excreta and all manner of animal entrails. But why?

Zoologists Konrad Lorenz and Desmond Morris maintain that we are driven to all this frenzied activity by the same elementary force that serves to ensure the continuation of the species: cosmetics are sexual triggers. But Robert Brain has argued that though women in the West wear make-up which is blatantly sexual, they are not communicating availability – they are merely following fashion. Western cosmeticizing is for social not sexual satisfaction.

In our increasingly visually-conscious world, we strain our imaginations for ever newer forms of beauty. It is all part of our instinctive urge to create. Yet for all our inventiveness some of the central images which drive this search are remarkably constant. Marilyn Monroe and Madonna, with white complexions, blue eyes and blonde hair, have carried on an ancient tradition of 'golden-goddess' beauty.

PALE AND INTERESTING

A dazzling white skin was rated as much more beautiful and infinitely more feminine than a swarthy one as far back as the middle ages. A fair complexion had other implicit advantages too. It hinted at a ladylike, even aristocratic life. Peasants who laboured in the fields could not aspire to such a delicate look: their skins – tanned from constant exposure to the weather – were regarded as coarse. And there was a further, more pressing reason for keeping the skin free from colour. A pale complexion distinguished the real ladies from those other 'ladies of the town'. Only prostitutes rouged.

So a well-born fourteenth-century lady, with her reputation to consider, kept behind the high walls of her castle and made sure that her face had little or no exposure either to sunshine or lively breezes. In addition, to gain instant pallor, she painted her face with white lead. It seemed the perfect finishing touch for achieving the palest, most aristocratic of complexions.

But was it? The paste that most women used was processed from vinegar, white of egg and white lead. The workers who made it fell ill with 'contorsion of the stomach, dizziness, shortness of breath and even blindness'.

And the cosmetic which was the end-product of their efforts was just as damaging for the women who used it. The only difference was that, for a little while, women were able to enjoy its spectacular effects before succumbing to its poisons.

Ceruse, as the basic mix was often called, came in different qualities. The finest, most expensive, and most sought-after was from Venice. It was also the one which contained the greatest amount of lead. British ceruses, which were generally adulterated with common whiting, were not good for the skin but they were less damaging than the heavily-leaded ones. Cosmetic snobbery, however, deplored the British ceruses and cherished the Venetian ones. Ceruse was a killer. The lead it contained was steadily and cumulatively absorbed into the body. And it corroded the skin. Yet women stubbornly continued to use it; it was so brilliantly white and so smooth and so very successful at hiding blemishes and filling in wrinkles and pock-marks. Men protested its dangers, but at the same time dearly loved those ravishingly white complexions.

Elizabeth I led the world with her 'ivory glow'. She used ceruse lavishly but needed progressively denser and denser applications as the lead ate more and more deeply into her skin. Towards the end of her life, she was using ceruse, so it was said, 'near half an inch thick'.

Even today and despite widespread knowledge of the dangers of lead, and legislation against using toxic ingredients or irritants in cosmetics, lead compounds have been found in boxes of low-cost colouring cosmetics from Taiwan. Marketed for children, they slipped into Britain under the brand names of Meyssa and Aroma Fashion Blenders. Their lead content was so high that they caused blisters and, in some children, brain damage. It is a sad fact that children absorb lead five times more easily than adults. One child suffered bouts of sickness and depression after using one of the kits. She lost weight, her face became pock-marked and her bottom lip became almost paralysed. Another victim suffered deterioration of her eyesight. After several such cases, alarms were sounded and the products called in.

But lead has proved to be only one of many aids to a paler complexion. High-spirited ladies in the sixteenth century did not stop at ceruse; they were prepared to 'swallow gravel, ashes, coal dust, tallow candles and for the nonce, labour and toil themselves to

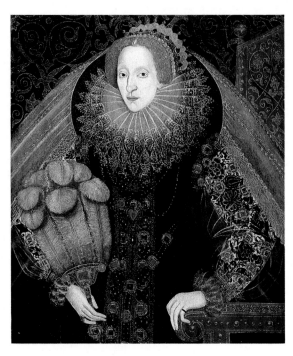

spoil their stomach, only to get a pale complexion', reported Michel de Montaigne. Another favourite recipe included sheep's trotters 'well chopped to get at the marrow'. In Denmark, a century later, the ladies pinned their faith in a cosmetic-wash known as 'Pigeon's Water', each bottle of which required seven or eight white pigeons plucked and minced.

But perhaps the most dangerous preparation of all came from Signora Toffana, who introduced seventeenth-century Italian ladies to a face preparation made from liquid arsenic. It produced many blanched faces but also, it seems, a great many widows. Six hundred Italian husbands were said to have been killed off – after intimate contact with the faces of their loved ones – before the Signora was arrested and executed. (Yet even in Victorian times, an arsenic soap was still being marketed.)

But most women remained stubbornly faithful to ceruse. One of the most famous and beautiful women of the eighteenth century, Maria, Lady Coventry, refused to be dissuaded from her addiction to white lead. Towards the end she kept the curtains of her bed drawn and refused to have a light in her room so that no one should see the terrible ravages of ceruse. She died when only twenty-seven.

Horace Walpole, in 1766, reported the fate of the pretty Lady Fortrose: 'killed like Lady Coventry and others, by white lead, of which nothing could break her'. And the following year, another beauty, the celebrated young actress and courtesan, Kitty Fisher, died from ceruse.

Men, who had also been using colourful cosmetics during the rumbustious days of the Restoration, suddenly took fright and became litigious about women and their foolish

ABOVE : An anonymous court painter's flattering view of the elderly, bewigged Elizabeth I
OPPOSITE : Elizabeth I (here portrayed by Glenda Jackson) used ceruse lavishly but needed progressively denser applications as the lead ate into her skin

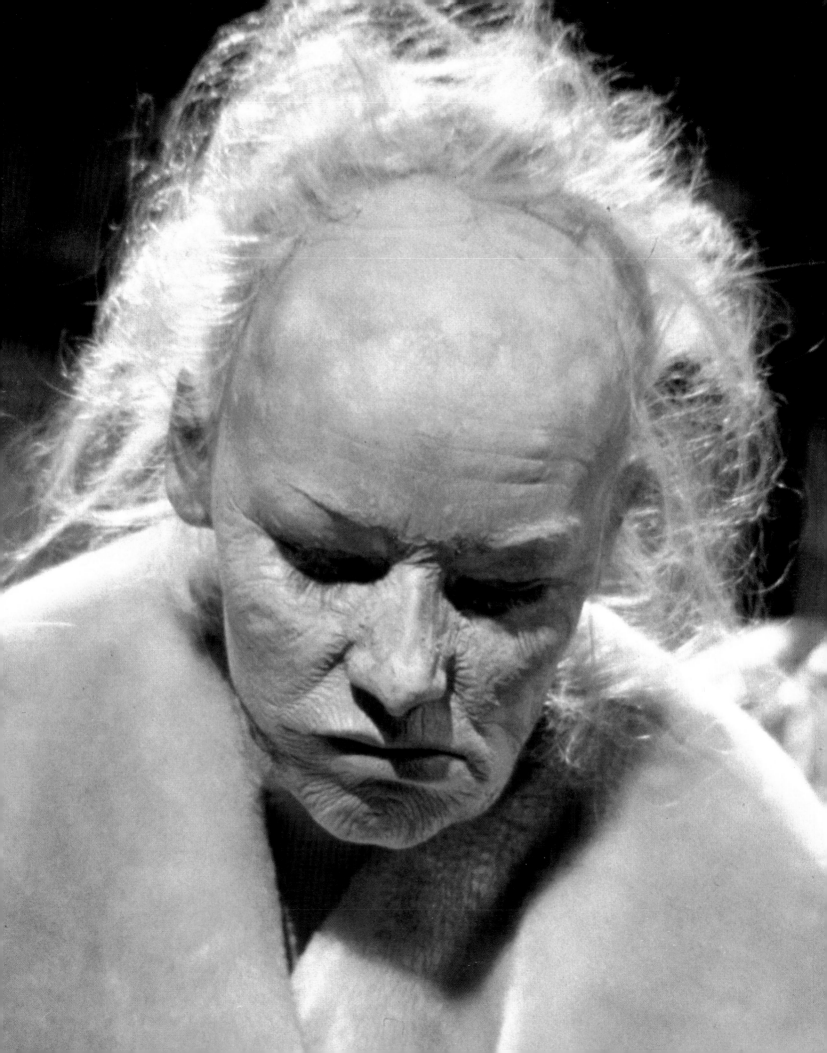

ways with cosmetics. They complained that they were being duped into marriage by the many 'artificial and deceiving aids' employed by women. One aggrieved husband wrote to *The Spectator* in 1711, more or less asking for his money back. Could the law intervene, he wondered, when a husband found that his wife was not the person he had intended to marry? He felt he had a case, because 'when she first wakes in a morning she scarce seems young enough to be the mother of her whom I carried to bed the night before. I shall take the liberty to part with her at the first opportunity, unless her father will make her portion suitable to her real, not her assumed countenance.'

An Act of Parliament to safeguard men was eventually passed in 1770, imposing the same penalties as for witchcraft. Though unenforcible, it did have a short-lived effect of discouraging some women from using cosmetics. And it probably did some good in hastening the end of the lethal ceruse.

By Queen Victoria's time florid gentlemen were putting perfumed chalk on their cheeks to tone down their colour, but Victorian ladies were under orders to remain totally innocent of artifice. So of course they bleached their skins in secret. Bottles of a substance known as Bloom were discreetly on sale though the product was known to have its own peculiar disadvantages. It masked and enamelled the face so thoroughly that attempts to wash with hot water merely cracked the brilliant white surface, and cold water ran off without disturbing it. And it certainly restricted any attempts at animated conversation. Over-excited speech, or any facial exertion, could fissure its surface with tiny, unbecoming cracks which looked suspiciously like wrinkles.

Nevertheless, determined ladies who wanted the mask-like favours of this complexion whitener were quite prepared to carry on with their 'blooming' in private – even though it meant remaining poker-faced in public.

Skin lighteners are still being used today with equally damaging effects, and for more serious social reasons: in an attempt to counteract racial prejudice. Merle Oberon fought all her life to keep her Eurasian origins a secret. At the height of her beauty she suffered from a terrible skin disease which left her scarred for the rest of her life. Just what caused her skin complaint remains unclear but her constant desire to whiten her dark skin was well known. And her use of 'toxic cosmetics' is recorded in Higham and Moseley's biography *Merle*.

There is no pill, so far, which will inhibit the production of melanin and change black skins to white. Hydroquinone, however, a powerful chemical capable of removing pigmentation from the skin will bleach out black patches in cases of vitiligo, a troublesome and distressing disturbance of the skin in which an underlying lack of melanin causes disfiguring white patches to appear on black skins. These patches are often so numerous that it is simpler to attempt to bleach the remaining black areas than re-pigment the white ones.

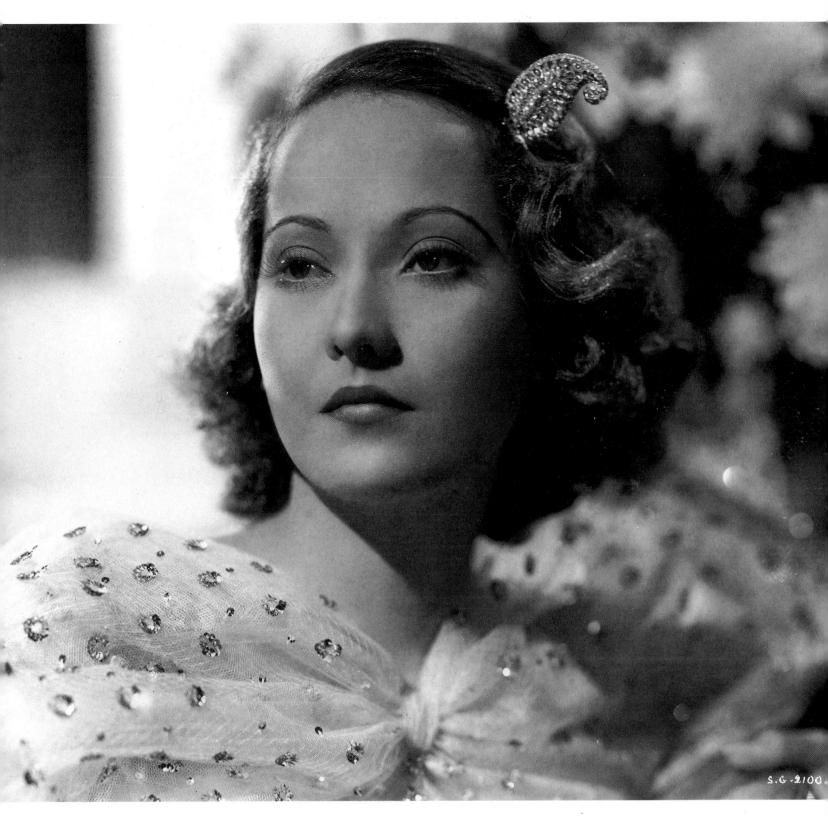

Merle Oberon fought all her life to keep her Eurasian origins a secret. By the end, her skin was badly scarred

In Britain, a leading chemist markets a product called Fade Out, useful for 'liver spots', which also contains hydroquinone. Dr Vernon Coleman, a popular writer on medical matters, has warned that the effect of hydroquinone is irreversible and not always pleasing. 'It is quite possible to produce "patchy" depigmentation and that can be nothing short of a cosmetic disaster. . . . I do not believe that any product containing hydroquinone should be bought over the counter since the effects can be very far reaching. If you want to try a permanent skin "bleach" then you should consult a doctor first.'

In South Africa an estimated 30 million packs of skin-lightening creams and lotions are sold each year – a market worth 20 million pounds. A number of lighteners are available. Some of these have been sold under the brand name of Softlite with product names like Superman Day Cream and Special. The active agent is hydroquinone and as many as 40% of black women in South Africa are now believed to be suffering from its effects.

Black domestic servants are especially vulnerable. According to Ms Ellen Kuzwayo, President of the Black Consumer Association, 'They think it is smart to be like Madam, with that white skin. The temptation to try these products seems quite irresistible. At first the results are encouraging, the skin certainly does bleach white. But then it turns dark and coarse and small black lumps appear under the surface. These grow larger and eventually merge with each other to create large, lumpy patches'. Dermatologist Dr Hilary Carman finds it difficult to understand women's obstinacy in continuing to use such products. 'They continue to buy creams when they know their friends' complexions are being devastated by the same creams.'

Mercury is another chemical which has its own history of disasters. Originally used to shape felt hats, it was found not only to bleach the skin of the workers but also to cause kidney and brain damage – hence the old expression 'mad as a hatter'. Yet until it attracted the attention of Health and Safety experts in 1985, a product called Roberts Medicated soap was still on sale in Britain. Its mercuric iodide content was said to cause sleeplessness, nausea, vomiting and kidney problems and even could be fatal. Banned in Britain, the soap still enjoys a good market overseas. Ladies, notably in Africa, continue to purchase it, in order to make their skin whiter. As TV Channel 4's *Bandung File* revealed, there are a number of these soaps containing mercury still available 'under the counter' and still being purchased by dark-skinned people who wish to make themselves paler. In June 1988 a member of parliament, Max Madden, called on the government to review once more the manufacture, sale and export of these products.

BLACK IS BEAUTIFUL

The cry, 'black is beautiful' was heard in the 1960s. But there was little in the huge range of cosmetics then on sale that was at all suitable for black skins. Successful groups like The Supremes with Diana Ross their star, did the best they could with scarlet or orange

NOTE Since going to press, we understand that the company manufacturing Roberts Medicated Soap does not now use any mercury compound in its soap.

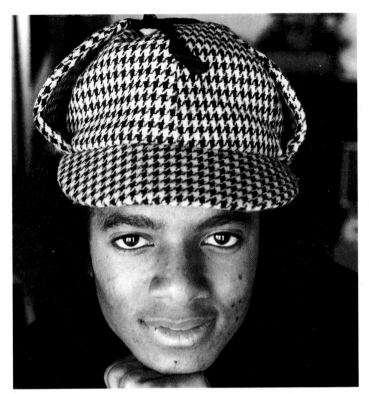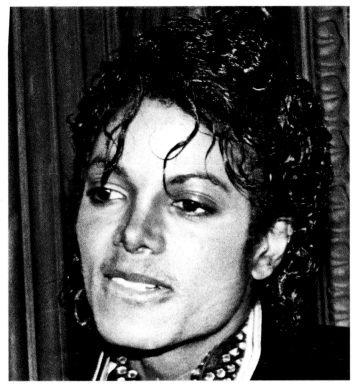

Is Michael Jackson's face falling apart? According to a Pretoria plastic surgeon, if transplanted bone does not knit properly, it will crumble, entailing yet more surgery

lipsticks and wigs of straight, European-style hair. Now, after the revolution, the picture has entirely changed. Black is unquestionably beautiful. Many fashionable Europeans have attempted to copy (not very successfully) Afro hair-styles and dreadlocks and traditional African styles, particularly in hair (see Ch. 8) which emphasise the sculpted look of the face, can be seen on many city streets.

But there is one black mega-star who evidently does not accept his natural colour, and who has, for the time being, outstripped all others in the risk-taking business of change: Michael Jackson. His skin has been bleached from black to near-white. After benefiting from much spectacular publicity about the cosmetic surgery responsible for the changes in his face, he now insists that all he has had are two nose jobs and a cleft put into his chin. But it is difficult to credit his new white skin and fined-down bone structure to a vegetarian diet. More credible are the observations of Michael's friends who say that when they commented he was looking pale and ill, he was unable to put things right by applying rouge. Extensive cosmetic surgery could have meant that make-up will no longer adhere to his skin. But 'hair of the dog' has become part of Michael's built-in lifestyle. Undeterred, they say that he immediately sought other means for adding colour to his face. And as soon as he discovered the answer he did not hesitate: he straightaway had his cheeks tattooed to give himself a permanently rosy glow.

THE LUST FOR BRONZE

Nowadays, a 'healthy' sun-tanned look is a 'must'. In spite of the widely-known dangers of developing cancer from the effects of the sun's rays, thousands upon thousands still flock to shadeless beaches for their annual grilling. Lying in row upon row in the blazing sun, they endure contorted postures, prickly heat, raw and peeling skin, mosquito bites . . . all in aid of that overall tan.

But chemists have now turned their attention to creating products which will produce a tan without the dubious benefits of ultra-violet exposure. In the beauty game when one dangerous pursuit has been recognised there is usually another waiting in the wings to take its place. From France has come the capsule Orobronze. Instructions are simple – swallow the pills, sit back, and you get tanned in a matter of days. And to make the tan permanent – just keep on taking the tablets.

There could be problems: the active ingredient in Orobronze is canthaxanthin, already widely used in fruit drinks, ketchups and soups. Unfortunately, canthaxanthin can cause interference with twilight vision and adaptation of the eye to the dark. An acceptable daily intake has, in fact, been defined by the World Health Organisation. In Orobronze, the daily recommended dose is less than one tenth of this maximum. But in the opinion of Dr George Mitchell, of the Welsh College of Medicine, '. . . who knows what this means over a length of time? Could it affect the kidneys . . . we just don't know. Other food colourings once considered safe are now banned. No way would I take it.'

In the United States, the Orobronze capsule is banned from public sale.

But for that successful look in an increasingly competitive world, and to maintain his desirability with women, modern man remains persuaded that a status-symbol tan is a 'must'. Two types of alternative 'bronzers' are available, the instant ones which will wash off at night and the chemical ones which develop on the skin. Advertisers have a cast-iron scientific and very seductive basis for their sales copy: the sun has become our enemy. Too much exposure can cause skin cancer. But, we are hastily assured, we must look tanned. So we must buy 'bronzers'.

PAINT POWER

Mary Quant noticed in the 1960s that, increasingly, we want to look pretty but with less bother. She experimented with a pill which would impart a healthy glow to the face, but eventually abandoned it. Who knows, perhaps such ideas were counter-productive to cosmetic sales?

In the days of Charles II, there were spirited cries for colour. For women, 'perfection' lay in a doll-like face of dazzling white topped with bright, well-rouged cheeks. Men, too, used cosmetics freely: the notorious hanging judge, Judge Jeffreys, was 'flagrant in his use of make-up'. There were, it is true, some men who expressed diffidence about the excessive use of rouge. Samuel Pepys, not at all averse himself to the pretty ladies, declared that he disliked to see a painted woman. Others, like the Earl of Chesterfield, considered women positively plain if they were without rouge. But the majority of sophisticated women at that time – and certainly those at Court – favoured the French influence: the ideal 'maquillage' was distinctly flamboyant. And, as ever, women were ready to try anything to achieve it.

A cosmetic known as 'Spanish Red' was popular for touching up the cheekbones. It consisted of powdered rouge liberally dispersed within a pad of hair and it looked remarkably like a modern pan scourer.

In the following century – the eighteenth – women added another cumulative poison to their already disastrous arsenal. Red lead became, for a while, a great favourite. Other paints containing poisonous heavy metals were popular too, though there were plenty of warnings about their dangers. In *The Art Of Preserving Beauty* (1754), Antoine Le Camus explained how brimstone and mercury could be reduced to a powder in a marble mortar which then: '. . . acquires so lively and so high a colour that it is called Vermilion. Some ladies mix it with paint wherewith they rub their cheeks, which is very dangerous for by using it frequently they may lose their teeth, acquire a stinking breath and excite a copious salivation.'

In Britain, rosy cheeks contrasting against pure white foreheads, necks and breasts, flourished up to the 1750s but began to decline in popularity as the century progressed. Just as in the fourteenth century, ladies of fashion suddenly began to avoid it, leaving only the prostitutes with their faces red.

Then it was the men's turn again: the 'Macaronis' arrived and, as dramatically as latter-day Punks, for some fifty years strutted the English scene with their brilliant, lavish make-up and elaborate coiffures. These 'Exquisites', ridiculous though they were, influenced fashion considerably.

In Greece at the time, those women who were still painting their cheeks pink became interested in a new product which was showing great promise. It was called Sulama and it not only reddened the cheeks, it also gave the skin a beautiful, porcelain-like gloss. But Sulama carried with it the awful risk of discovery. Any curious or jealous companion – by deliberately chewing on a clove and then breathing on the lady's face – could test his suspicions: one puff and the lady's cheeks would turn yellow.

The French continued to redden their cheeks long after British ladies had put away their rouge pots altogether. By 1781 French women were using two million pots of rouge a year. According to Horace Walpole: 'Any woman in Paris who neglected to wear rouge was assumed to be English.' He might well have added 'or a prostitute' for whilst fashionable Parisiennes in the late eighteenth century were sporting chalk-white faces and flaming red cheeks, French prostitutes tried to distinguish themselves with a natural look. This of course was entirely contrary to the British fashion and must have confused many a globe-trotting gentleman.

The rouges at that time were usually made from poisonous metallic compounds. Even the 'least injurious of these' according to one report, 'has caused tremblings of the muscles of the face, ending in paralysis'. Some of these heavy metal preparations also had the embarrassing trick of reacting with vapours in the air. The sulphur from a coal fire, for example, might easily change pink cheeks to black.

In early Victorian times, just as in the days of the Macaronis and the lusty days of Charles II, men were not averse to using cosmetics. Those with ruddy faces quietened them down with pale powders whilst those who were excessively pallid added colour to their cheeks. And this cast no slur on their masculinity. Lord Malmesbury was skilfully rouged, but Disraeli vouched for his manliness. 'In fact,' said Mr Disraeli, 'the two most manly persons I ever knew, Palmerston and Lyndhurst, both rouged'.

Victorian women still hankered after a white skin, though the unhealthy-looking pallor associated with the 'green sickness' was frowned upon. This all-too-common anaemic condition was understood to be brought about by tight lacing. Afflicted women, swooning from over-compression and with faces strangely livid, tried secretly to coax just a little, natural-looking colour into their grey/green faces. Schnouda, a newly-invented liquid rouge made from the chemical, alloxan, became popular but it was difficult to judge precisely when it would begin to take effect and just how intense the colour would be once it had been applied. Fine judgement, restraint, and a good deal of practice were required for successful results. The penalty – and the shame – for the heavy-handed novice was the embarrassment of red cheeks suddenly flaring and colouring up at some quite inopportune moment. And as many a Victorian woman came to realise, a guilty reddening of the cheeks from Schnouda could never be passed off as a maidenly blush.

The wheel of fashion keeps turning full circle. Verushka – the Sixties model girl in Antonioni's film *Blow Up* – decorated her face with stripes and patterns as bold as any Papuan chieftain's. Stencilled and painted with fantasy flowers of unlikely colours – the extraordinary designs on her face and body were a foretaste of the dazzling displays which were to follow in the Punk and Rock music world of the 1970s. Even so, in the early 1980s pop-singer Toyah Willcox with rainbow-painted face and hair fanned out to peacock proportions, still came as something of a shock. Yet the psychedelic artwork of Toyah's face, drawn from a palette of safer, twentieth-century cosmetic products, has more than a little in common with the wild and spectacular attempts of Nero's wife Poppaea. She worked hard at being beautiful, covering her face with white lead, brilliant purple-red 'fucus' (the deadly poison made from mercury) for her cheeks and lips and black antimony for her eyelids. To complete the picture she used bright blue paint for emphasising her breast-veins and pumice-stone for polishing her teeth.

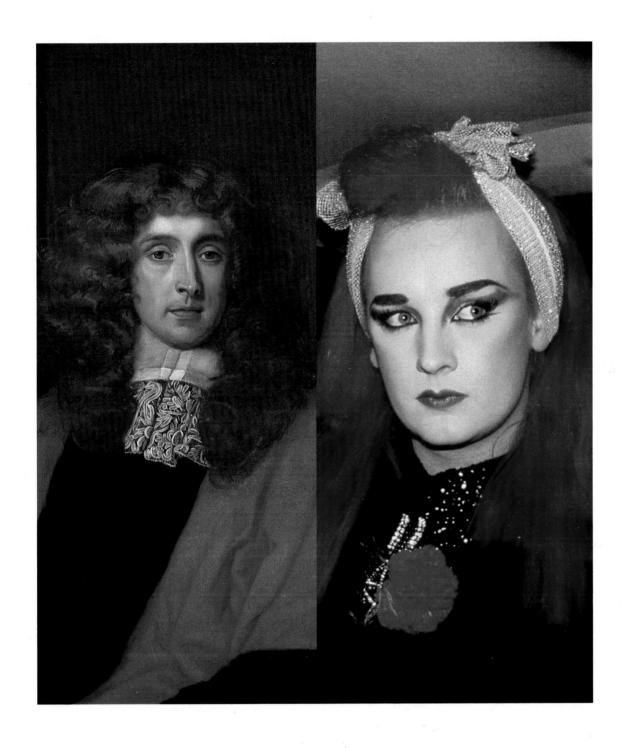

L E F T : Seventeenth-century Judge Jeffreys, notorious for his brutality, was
'flagrant in his use of make-up'

R I G H T : Boy George. Uninhibited bursts of colour on male faces throw us into
a sort of piquant confusion about gender

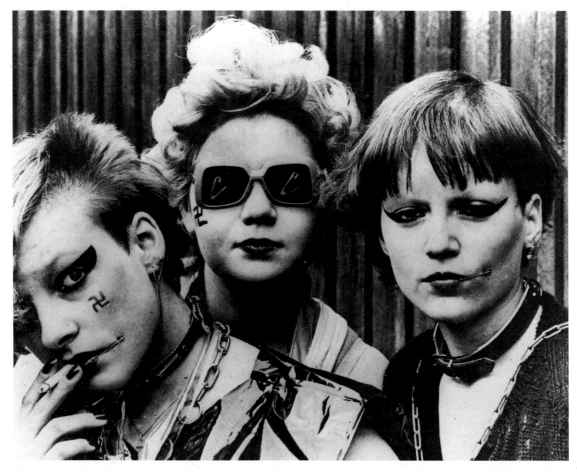

Almost two thousand years later, and as from another planet, came the Punks, with cox-combs of coloured hair, painted faces and trappings of leather and chain. The dictionary suggests that 'Punks' are worthless foolish people who are miserable. In reality they may not always have been miserable, but it is true that the message of the Punks was a desperate one – no future. And there was little they felt they could do save make their protest – through the medium of their clothes, their make-up and above all, their hair.

Some festooned their faces with threatening symbols – razor-blades, chains and studs. Pallid-white make-up – a frequent choice – was intensified by the contrast of heavy mascara and fearsome designs around the eyes. Tattoos were popular. Names and messages were engraved on necks, shaven skulls, cheekbones. Menacing chains rattled from ear to nose; hair colours were psychedelic and dazzling. But true Punk style required individuality. Black leather might be crisp and clean, or battered and baggy – better still, half and half. And such personalised dressing could be highly therapeutic. Life feels all the better for individual self-expression.

Although the Punk movement is more or less defunct in Britain, Punk culture is spreading in countries such as Poland – perhaps because other independent organisations

A B O V E : Punk style contrasted pallid make-up with heavy mascara are banned. Young people are powerfully attracted to this more colourful kind of protest. Polish Punks live for the moment. The vision of a nuclear holocaust in the not too distant future is too dreadful to contemplate. Their make-up, coloured hair, ritualistic gear, offers a kind of temporary protection. If they were asked about what happens when a Punk starts getting on in years, no doubt they would give the same answer as one young man from Yorkshire, 'I don't think I'll live long enough to grow old.'

Today's hunger for sensation has led some men into wild cosmetic excursions. But this is no real novelty: Henri III used to walk the streets of Paris 'made up like an old coquette'. And those eighteenth-century dandies, the Macaronis, weighed down in enormous elaborate wigs and wearing just as much powder as their wives and mistresses, created an impression not unlike David Bowie in the Seventies and Boy George in the Eighties. In today's world of popular music, colours that dazzle and designs that shock are essential and indispensable. Songs are not just sung any more, they are 'performed'. Fans are buying more videos to look at and fewer records just for the sound. The uninhibited bursts of colour on male faces throw us into a sort of piquant confusion about gender. Sexual ambiguity has been recognised by pop-stars for what it is – a guaranteed attention-getter making us all think harder about masculinity and femininity. In 1973, Bowie – appearing as the character Aladin Sane – seemed outrageous. What was disconcerting was that his make-up was no longer simply theatrical and part of the act – he wore it out-and-about, and seriously. In doing so, he was giving us our first taste of pop androgyny. Later on, having caught the popular imagination, he could afford to look more conservative, even conventional, though always open to change. He keeps us guessing. Boy George continues where Bowie's Aladin Sane left off – startling and delighting fans with innovative make-up and dress, and untroubled by any rigid dividing line between male and female. Quite deliberately, the mysterious fascinations of ambiguity are being used as powerful weapons in the battle for popular attention.

5. THE FACE:
CHANGING THE TEXTURE

PLANING AND PLUMPING

The skin is often referred to as a 'third kidney' because of its excretory functions. It sloughs off dead skin cells and generally serves as an exit route for worn-out tissue so that the complexion may bloom afresh. Within its topmost layer – or epidermis – cells reproduce, then travel to the surface, die, and eventually are shed. The process takes about a month. But there is a snag. This shedding process slows down with age, often causing the complexion to become muddy and sallow. But the difficulty has not gone unnoticed. Three major therapeutic methods have been devised to deal with the complexion's recalcitrant debris.

The first is known as 'Resurfacing Therapy'. It achieves its purpose – often with the use of strong chemicals such as phenol – by peeling off the surface of the skin. A second alternative method, known as 'Dermabrasion', does the same job in precisely the way its name suggests – by abrading the offending epidermis in a kind of surgical 'sandpapering' or planing, using electrically powered instruments not unlike the wire brushes of a household power tool. Depth of excavation is critical: over-zealous penetration can leave very bad scarring and uneven patches of skin colour – which is why surgeons in New York are trying out computers carefully programmed to a precise duration time and depth.

For the less adventurous, there are plenty of 'exfoliant' creams available now which provide a gritty lather when wetted. Colloquially known as 'scruffers' and 'skin polishers' they will scour the skin effectively though much less vigorously.

For plumping up skin rather than planing it, there is another system: Beneath the epidermis lies the true, living skin with its elaborate warp and weft of fibres made up mostly of the important protein collagen. It is this 'network' of fibres which gives the skin so much of its resilience. Because of illness, lack of vitamins, exposure to sun, or even through heredity the fibres may become disorganised. When this happens, the delicate network is disturbed, so changing the shape of the dermis, and the epidermis is no longer such a snug fit. So it sags, collapses into any convenient crack, and a wrinkle is born. The aim of modern cosmeticians has been to reorganise the distressed fibres by ingeniously creating replacement collagen and attempting to feed it to them.

But only by surgery using so-called collagen implants can this be achieved. Attempts at replacement by simply massaging collagen-rich moisturiser creams into the surface of the skin have met with scepticism. Malcolm Greaves, Professor of Dermatology at St John's Hospital, London, is dismissive of most rejuvenating creams. He maintains that although they may plump up the skin for a few hours by hydrating it, they have little or no permanent effect. 'The best and most simple way to have a youthful skin is to avoid sun, exposure and extremes of heat and cold,' he says.

What is often not made clear in advertising copy is that moisturising creams work by providing a barrier to prevent moisture loss; they do not add moisture, they simply prevent moisture getting out.

There have been other criticisms. One cellular anti-ageing cream, on sale in the 1980s for £55 per tiny pot, carried with it the name of a well-known heart surgeon. But as Carmel Fitzsimmons pointed out, the sheep's grease (lanolin) it contained is known to be a common cause of skin allergies.

One anti-wrinkle cream, Retin-A, has been tested in the United States at Boston University School of Medicine and results pronounced promising. In the University Hospital of Wales a pilot study has also shown promising results but experts agree, it is early days for this anti-ageing cream: tests are now being designed for any side effects. Since Vitamin A acne preparations have already been linked with birth defects, the use of Retin-A by pregnant women is unlikely to be recommended.

More natural ways have been sought out. Liz Tilberis, editor of *Vogue*, believes strongly in drinking plenty of plain water. The makers of Volvic water encourage this too, but their water comes in bottles and is somewhat more expensive than water from the tap. It is, they say, mineral water of unusual purity straight from the Auvergne and 'filtered through alternate layers of fine porous rocks and hard volcanic stone'. But once again, moderation is called for. Water intoxication is a real and dangerous disorder. *The British Medical Journal* recently reported the case of a man who found comfort is swilling water over an aching tooth. He swallowed, according to his wife, 'a bathful of water' after which he became unconscious and needed hospitalisation. Doctors now believe that it is possible to swallow enough water to kill you – and without any warning sign that it is time to stop.

Washing the face with soap and water is deplored by most cosmetic houses who recommend instead cleansing lotions followed by hydrating creams. Others seem not to be so sure – a water-jet bath and a 'space age computerised bath to get rid of dead face cells of skin' have both had their moments. One woman's magazine in 1979 declared excitedly that women were 'rediscovering the power of water' and gave the reassuring news that 'there is no harm in using water on your face'. At one salon in London in the same year, even the mighty oceans were called in to assist. A 'sea soap facial' with 'deep sea kelp cleanser sea spray' was offered, topped up with a genuine 'sea mud pack'.

In fact, the cosmetic world seems to resurrect – even divine – water once a decade. In April 1988 the magazine *Best* featured 'The Wonder of Water' declaring it to be 'calorie free' and well worth drinking. And a good way of increasing the circulation, they said, was to 'fill a bath with cold water and with a T-shirt on to keep you warm, step into it and walk on the spot for one minute. Afterwards put on a pair of warm socks.'

But there is strong competition for these spa-like, back-to-nature trends. As we approach the twenty-first century, techniques to enhance our beauty become ever more sophisticated. Biotherm has designed a machine to diagnose the actual 'biological age' of the skin, which might of course be alarmingly greater than its actual age, while the Bioscope will take an imprint of your skin on a slide, and then unkindly project a magnified image of it on to a screen. From Japan, Shiseido's Skin Imaging Computer will allow a latex replica of the skin to be taken, magnified and paraded on a screen. Lancôme have produced an electronic probe which will look beneath the skin's surface to determine its moisture content. Yet another machine measures firmness and elasticity with a suction tube. Results are uncompromisingly signalled on a visual display unit. Helena Rubinstein – also preoccupied with moisture in the skin – uses another hydration-reading electronic probe.

Again, there is a snag. As modern interior designers have already discovered, kitchens as sterile as NASA laboratories need humanising with a pretend fire, baskets of logs and the presence of a friendly old tabby cat. The human touch is lacking. An 'Image Analyser' from Elizabeth Arden could scan the craters of the skin by light beam and then – aided by an input of further information from the customer – produce a print-out giving a detailed profile of skin type, accompanied by product recommendations. But alas, it could not talk, and soon was relegated to join near-relations on the scrap-heap of cosmetic gimickry.

And what of the validity of claims made by the makers of skin-improvers? What, if any, is the objective scientific evidence? Conscientious cosmetic firms have been doing their best to establish proof. Promises of specific improvement have been put to the test. Revlon have designed a skin-evaluation test in which tape is applied to the cheek, forehead and neck immediately before and then ten days after using one of their products. Visible differences in skin texture are then assessed. Professor Ronald Marks at the University Hospital of Wales has developed an extensometer which will monitor the elasticity of the skin – before and after treatment.

And modern research insists that there is indeed some virtue in attempting to rehabilitate the skin with creams during the night. One of the explanations offered is that the cellular chemistry responsible for growth and repair is accelerated during sleep and therefore has 'a higher energy charge'. All sorts of hi-tech methods are becoming available to analyse, store and call up at will, all available information on the present biological status and recent development of a particular man or woman's complexion.

The Advertising Standards Authority in Britain has a code of practice for the writing of advertising copy. If an advertiser makes a very direct claim about the ageing process then he must be able to prove that his product works in that way.

Any cosmetics which suggest they have a more fundamental effect are no longer – by definition – cosmetics. They have become drugs and must comply with the 1968 Medicines Act. Have anti-ageing creams crossed the line between cosmetics and drugs?

Recently, the DHSS and the DTI instructed nine companies to conduct tests to see if certain creams can cause cancer on animals' skins.

In America the FDA has gone further. Twenty-two companies have been warned that if they make anti-ageing claims for their creams then they must provide scientific evidence for this and also provide evidence for their safety. Alternatively, they should drop claims that they can reverse ageing or that they can bring about any basic underlying changes in the skin. After a year of wrangling, the phrases 'anti-wrinkle' and 'anti-ageing' have been forbidden; in their place advertisers now say 'smoothes wrinkles' and 'improves the surface of the skin'.

And there is a further problem, as Professor Greaves points out. If, as advertisers claim, these creams really are stimulating cell renewal and cell division, what will be their long-term effect – especially on skins already damaged by over-exposure to sunlight?

SOFTENING UP THE MALE

Fifty years ago, a man would lather his face, strop his razor and remove his stubble, as a daily duty. It was the sum total of his dedication to his face. Exceptionally, he might let the barber provide him with a faint whiff of eau-de-cologne. On special occasions, there might be a two-minute pat with some gift-wrapped after-shave, or even a tentative adventure with his wife's new perfumed talc. But nothing more fancy. A business executive gave himself a little more licence, from time to time submitting himself to hygienic treatments designed to clear his skin of impurities. A hot towel and steam treatment lasted thirty minutes or so and often took place in the bowels of one of the city's more expensive hotels. But he did it – so he said – for relaxation and the opportunity to meet and talk with colleagues – it had nothing to do with beauty. Everyone knew that only the theatrical, the deviant and those whose duties involved public appearances wore make-up, or would dream of confessing to time-consuming rituals to better their complexions.

Nowadays there are plenty of men who are prepared to spend every bit as much time as women do on the rejuvenation of their faces. Though prejudice against rouge and lipstick has not completely disappeared, scenting, creaming and toning the complexion are seen as proper activities for the modern man.

The changes came about gradually: in 1923 the correct and traditional toiletry gift for men was the Gentleman's Casket, a no-nonsense box which housed a sterilised brush, stick of shaving soap, solid brilliantine and a cake of transparent soap. It was produced by Pears. Twenty years later, during the war, American servicemen had become so used to receiving gift packs of more tempting toiletries that they were growing quite blasé about using face powder – which they preferred to call talc; and face cream – which they called massage cream. The idea spread. By 1964, even Eskimo gentlemen who normally plucked their beards out with pliers twice a year were becoming interested in something a little more sophisticated. Cosmetic houses were triumphant. 'Make-up for men is here,' cried Fabergé's Paul D. Blackman. But . . . 'Just don't call it make-up'. So The Gentleman's Casket and its cohorts quietly disappeared, and in their place came robust, virile, manly products calling themselves Waterloo, Tycoon, Gravel, Brut. And who more convincing than an ex-boxer to sanction their use? (Yet who could have anticipated that, in 1987, Fabergé would report sales of 12 million items from the Brut range?)

Attention spread to other bodily parts. Men with a secret taste for make-up were encouraged to come out of their closets. Executives in Madison Avenue began to have their hair waved and their eyebrows tinted.

And so the 'New Man' was born – a trendy dresser, smooth-skinned, slim, discreetly made up, hair styled at a salon. He was certainly not averse to trying out more caring treatments for his face. He even ventured into beauty parlours hitherto monopolised by women. And he eventually found his way into those advanced hi-tech clinics where science has sold its soul to beauty. Here, he has begun to feel surprisingly at home. Because the beauty world is changing. Increasingly computerised and heavy with quasi-scientific jargon and gadgetry many of its rituals and recommendations now come in such scientific guise that the hesitant male on the threshold of beauty culture is quite reassured. Attending to his face – but to an accompaniment of laboratory language – seems somehow more acceptable, less feminine, less embarrassing. Very shortly he will be throwing off inhibitions altogether: soon he will be reading print-outs on complexion care as eagerly as he reads motor-car manuals and catalogues of drill-bits.

Commerce has caught the trend and has been quick to encourage it. Women's beauty magazines carry supplements for the male. Cosmetic houses are ready with beautifiers which could just as easily be 'his' as 'hers'. The male who remains backwardly diffident about all this is being catered for too. He is being gently humoured by advertising carefully chiselled for the old masculine stereotypes. Magazines parade macho men straight from an oil-rig or even a battlefield, with suggested cosmetic products strapped to their protective helmets. In a discreet black booklet, Aramis confide to men 'Why Your Face Shows Stress'. Hard days and long nights take their toll, they say, 'so does pollution, enclosed working spaces, lack of fresh air, noise and air travel'. This is why they have 'bio-engineered', in their Aramis Lab Series, skin-saving products which include Razor Burn Relief – 'a unique therapy for post-shave discomfort'. Their products for men are not marketed as beautifiers, they are survival aids to combat weather-abused or office-bound skin, stress and manly fatigue.

Guérlain are now marketing face powder for men. Called 'Terracotta' it comes in two shades and with the option of an applicator strongly resembling a shaving brush. The brush costs almost as much as the powder. The British firm of Land and Burr now markets

Odalisque perfume for men in a pewter flask. There is no shortage of advice, no lack of ingenuity, no absence of new ideas in this ever-increasing beauty-culture business once so aptly described as 'the industry without a recession'.

URINE – THE ULTIMATE IN RECYCLING

Urine has long been recognised as having beautifying properties. Chinese ladies have, for centuries, especially favoured drinking the urine of young males. Today, in the West, enthusiasts explain that the valuable minerals and salts it contains are capable of curing many kinds of sickness and disease. Applied externally, urine packs, they say, can heal skin disorders, burns and wounds and can soothe sunburn. On the battlefield, *in extremis*, urine has been shown to be a serviceable, first-aid medication.

This versatile waste product is – perhaps surprisingly – completely sterile. Infinitely more refined than the substantial face-packs of crocodile dung so favoured by the Ancient

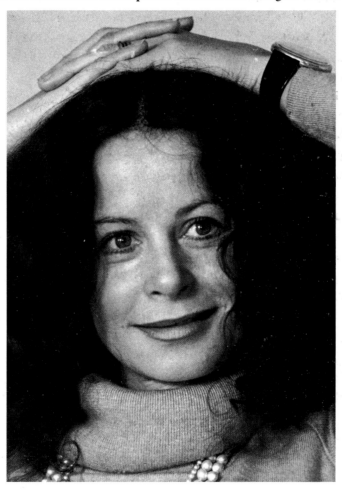

Actress Sarah Miles, practitioner of urine therapy – the ultimate in recycling

Egyptians, though perhaps not quite so pleasant as the milk baths which Cleopatra believed in, it has many practical advantages. It is cheap! And it is readily available. From a healthy donor its smell should not be too unpleasant. As for its flavour, devotees, already convinced of its powers, insist that it simply tastes of whatever the owner has recently been drinking or eating. It does have one disadvantage though – it tends to decompose fairly quickly and therefore most of its advocates advise using it before it takes on the qualities of a vintage brew.

In Britain, urine therapy does not have the unqualified approval of the medical profession. There is, however, one flourishing treatment centre which uses it – in Hertfordshire – run by an osteopath from Canada.

In California, the urine cult is more popular. Actress Sarah Miles is one dedicated believer and consumer. She found her faith in urine after attending a therapy clinic in Los Angeles where the therapist injected her own urine back into her own body. Said Sarah: 'They were very expensive injections, considering the stuff comes free.' And it was her own, anyway.

But she is a confirmed believer. And she no longer needs expensive injections. Instead, she simply drinks her own urine every day and finds that the taste is not 'too awful', though she admits she does prefer to take her daily dose with apple juice. 'I don't just drink it either,' she adds. 'I also wipe it on my face and use it to heal cuts and sores.'

There are plenty of others who share her enthusiasm. Urine is still widely used in the East. A brisk, mainly appreciative correspondence in Indian newspapers followed the public declaration by Prime Minister Desai that he regularly drank his urine for his health. But not all Indians agree that it is beneficial. In *The Indian Express* of December 1978, Dr Abraham Paul declared that since hormones in urine were killed by digestive juices, the liquid is useless when drunk. He conceded, however, that the traditional Ayurvedic physicians claimed beneficial results from the external application of urine: they believed it to be useful in curing eczema and other skin diseases. And not so very long ago, a folk remedy for sunburn was to press the damp portion of a baby's nappy against burning cheeks.

But most of us have a natural revulsion to drinking a waste product which is, when all is said and done, excreta. After all, Nature has gone to a lot of trouble in designing our bodies to get rid of it. It seems perverse to ingest it again. Its alleged advantages need to be carefully weighed against any possible damaging effects.

The Japanese have investigated more closely the possible utility of urine, but they have found practical problems. In *The Japan Times* in 1965, a new, urine-based drug was declared to be effective in dissolving blood clots, but with the disadvantage that a copious 50 litres of germ-free urine were needed to produce each remedial shot: a daunting production problem for its commercial exploiters.

Three hundred years ago, when it was not so easy to dispose rapidly of mankind's constant flow, urine was harvested in quantity and recipes for its beauty-enhancing use were naturally enough followed. One seventeenth-century book, *Artificiall Embellishments of Arts Best Directions* overflowed with ideas. One of its recipes recommended that 'ladies wishing to repair the beauty of an itching or scabby skin' should, 'Take as much man's urine as will serve to bathe the diseased up to the knees; add thereto charcoal or oak powdered and black hellebore. . . .' Used for fifteen mornings or longer if required, this method was said to have a highly beneficial effect on all parts of the body. It would prove a general cure-all for every skin complaint, 'whether it be tetter, leprosy, itch or running scab'.

PIGEON'S BLOOD AND VITRIOL

Artificiall Embellishments of Arts Best Directions was the best-selling beauty book of 1665. It was full of exciting advice and was enthusiastically in favour of urine. Its author, J. Jeamson, was a man blessed with the gift of delivering the unseemly, the unpleasant and the downright bizarre in language so lyrical and confident that even the most nervous and least experimental of ladies must have been totally disarmed. He urged his readers to: 'prize the medicines commended to you in this chapter as rarities; they'll make the hills and dales of uneven faces meet, levelling them to such a smoothness that little Cupid, though blind, may sport himself there and never stumble.'

Spots, he said, should be anointed with 'powdered pigeon's dung, flax-feed and French barley, all soaked in strong vinegar'. However, to cure redness and fiery pimples, he really did prefer 'blood-letting . . . chiefly in the median vein, in both the arms, some days being interposed: then in the vein of the forehead, afterwards the neck.' Again, 'You may apply leeches to the cheeks and chin to evacuate the blood that is amassed under the skin.' Alternatively, 'Spread on the visage the warm blood of a pigeon, pullet or capon drawn newly from under their wings; let the blood lay on all night; in the morning wash it off with warm water or the decoction of soap, oatmeal or the like, or take fresh flesh of a neck of beef, veal or mutton, cut two or three thin slices, lay them on the red places and change them often, or else they will stink.'

A century after Mr Jeamson's advices, fluid beautifiers were once again preoccupying women. One face-wash, popular for more than twenty years, was launched in 1775 with a quite spectacular splash: 'Take 5 quarts of brandy,' began the recipe. 'Add frankincense, gum arabic, mastic, benjamin, cloves, nutmeg, pinenuts, sweet almonds and musk, all bruised and distilled,' and you would then have created a versatile product known as 'Imperial Water', which promised to 'take away wrinkles and render the skin extremely delicate; it also whitens the teeth and abates the toothache, sweetens the breath and strengthens the gums. Foreign ladies prize it highly.'

A more radical approach came from the Duchess of Newcastle, and involved skin-stripping: much better to excavate for a fresh new surface underneath, having first removed all the unwanted old skin with oil of vitriol (concentrated sulphuric acid – much stronger than battery acid).

This kind of skin-stripping held few fears for determined women in the eighteenth century. Lady Mary Wortley Montagu 'applied muriatic [hydrochloric] acid 60% strong' to her face. After a long week of suffering from slow cautery, she was satisfied to find that her friends considered her complexion 'fashionably improved' even though 'an attack of typhoid fever would have been a less dangerous and more effective means of attaining her end'.

Lady Mary, a renowned traveller and social leader of her day, had a vigorous experimental approach to life. She had already suffered considerably from the effects of another cosmetic known as Balm of Mecca – a product much sought-after by ladies in Britain who had heard wonderful reports from abroad about its beautifying properties. She had tried it during her travels in Turkey, but was so shocked by its disastrous effects that she wrote a warning to ladies at home: 'the next morning . . . my face was swell'd to be a very extraordinary size. It remained in this lamentable stage three days during which you may be sure I pass'd my time very ill.'

In 1911 in the United States, a poisonous cosmetic called Klintho Cream, which contained mercury, was banned by the government. But the resourceful makers simply removed the words 'absolutely harmless' from its label and back it came on the market. One physician made matters worse by prescribing iodide of potash for a victim's severely inflamed face. This reacted with the mercury in the cream and the unfortunate face flared into a brilliant vermilion. A second physician hurriedly called in to the emergency prescribed sulphur ointment which, in contact with the mercury, turned the skin quite black.

At about the same time in Britain electrical treatments were all the rage. In 1909 the Davis Electric Medical Battery was bruited as the greatest invention of the century. It promised to 'destroy old age microbes' and make the blood go 'leaping, bounding, tingling' through the body. A beaming young woman plugged into an electric socket advertised its powers.

Even more desperate were the efforts of the Countess of Thanet's mother, an eighteenth-century lady who evidently believed love-making to be the greatest stimulant to beauty. This resolute old lady remained unshakeable in her determination to enjoy the therapeutic benefits of a vigorous love-life. When her husband finally succumbed to fatigue – if we are to believe the report of an English parson – she sought out a young man and having proved his talents, she promptly killed him. She then fed the distilled remains of this once-virile youth to her ageing husband in an attempt to revive his flagging, amorous energies. The parson seems to have kept the result a secret.

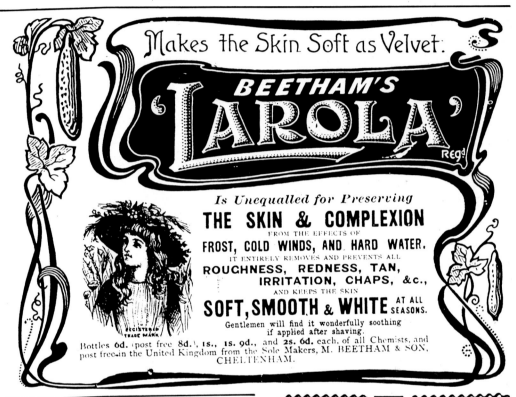
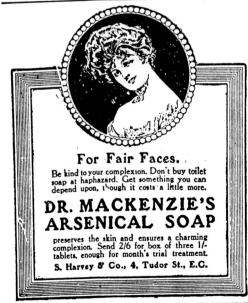

During pious Victorian times water had the sort of spell of popularity it periodically enjoys in the twentieth century. A woman of fifty who was reported as having the skin of a young girl, said that her secret was . . . she always washed in hot water. But one of her friends, equally blessed, stole her thunder by insisting that her way was better – she washed first with hot water but then followed with cold, 'in the Russian fashion'. Another said she personally preferred washing with hot water in the morning and cold at night. A nineteenth-century magazine, daring for its day, eclipsed them all and said 'Wash in wine!' But it had to be the right wine. Blondes should always employ a good Rhine wine and brunettes a Medoc. The complexion was fussy about this. In other quarters, enormous kettles, blankets and intricate arrangements of pipes were set up to provide steam baths for those ladies who preferred their water in more penetrating form.

All in all, perhaps the Countess of Thanet's belief in love as the supreme beautifier was not so far out after all. Film star Ursula Andress is certainly at one with the Countess. 'Love making is the greatest stimulant to beauty,' she says. Joan Collins agrees, 'Sex is one of the cheapest of all beauty treatments.' However, she does not accept that looks are the be-all and end-all of a woman's life and so she is against cosmetic surgery, saying she has never had any performed on her. Into her mid-fifties now, she works out with weights for about fifteen minutes a day in her personal gym, and does 50 sit-ups and 25 push-ups a day. Talitha Getty is more cautious, 'with a good man you don't need beauty treatments . . . not at first!' That sex is good for beauty is almost certainly true. The body's hormonal system, stimulated by sexual activity, should produce beneficial effects on the skin. And as the female sex hormones decline in the fifties, there is always the possibility of supplementing them with HRT (Hormone Replacement Therapy), though the considerable benefits of this must be balanced against any carcinogenic side-effects which some say may be associated with it.

CUTTING AND CARVING

While Westerners, for generations, have been investing time and money in resurfacing their faces to make them smoother, other cultures have been furrowing exotic patterns into theirs. Cutting into the surface of the flesh – both of the face and the body – to create scars has always been especially popular among peoples with dark skin. Fortunately for them, the desire for colour can easily be satisfied because the scars have the advantage of revealing the brightly coloured flesh beneath.

But introducing colour as an aesthetic novelty is by no means the primary reason for the practice of scarification: its major purpose has more often been to indicate who you are and what you are. These highly-defined patterns can accurately place an individual in a specific group. Social status, too, can be carved into the skin: royalty can be recognised in

OPPOSITE ABOVE: Ursula Andress: 'Love-making is the greatest stimulant to beauty'

OPPOSITE BELOW: For some African girls scarring commenced at puberty and was repeated and elaborated every few years

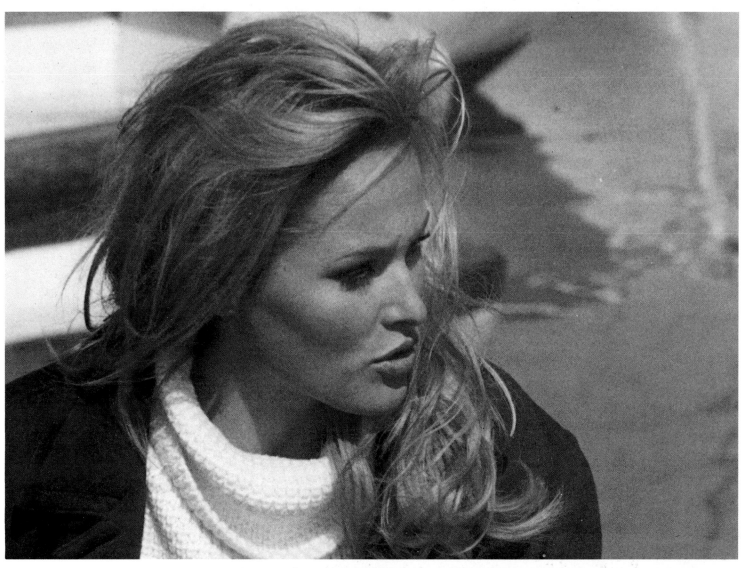

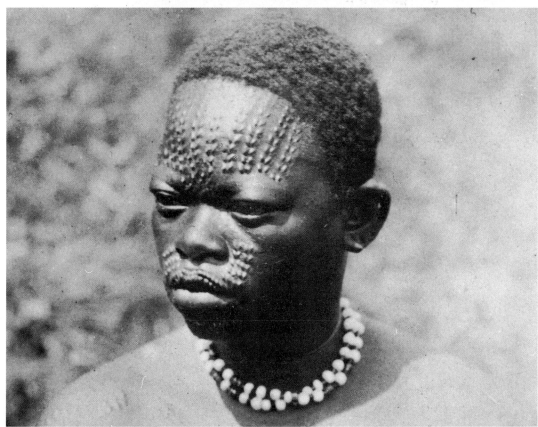

this way. Important events may also be recorded by notching the flesh of face and body with appropriate markings.

But most of all, scarring has been used to signal successful passage through important initiation rites. Boys in West Africa often received their first facial scarification at puberty. Then – since their personality must inevitably change as they progress to maturity – further decoration was necessary. Scratching, as well as repeated cutting of an old scar – though intensely painful – fulfilled this need. It raised the skin tissue higher and higher, and in this way physically echoed the boy's psychological development. Similarly, the scarification of Nuba girls from Southern Sudan was used to mark their physiological progress: scarring commenced at puberty and was repeated and elaborated every few years.

Very often, deliberate mutilation of the face has been used to indicate sorrow and mourning. In ancient Greece and Rome – and until it was forbidden by law – women tore at their cheeks with their fingernails to display grief. Sometimes scarification was religious, its aim being to show that a proper relationship with the gods and the spirits had now been established.

But whatever the motive, carving the skin and flesh beneath cannot fail to be intensely painful, especially when the instruments used are unsophisticated. In New Guinea, they still use a hooked thorn first of all to lift up the skin before slicing it with a razor; the higher the skin can be raised before cutting, the more dramatic will eventually be the scar. The Abipone people of South America also used sharp thorns and a mixture of blood and ashes to produce high weals – a distinctive mark of their clan. And they continued to enlarge these by carving deeper and deeper and then stuffing wads into the cuts to encourage the flesh to stand up.

Mutilation in this way is rare in the West, but not entirely unknown. Scar marks indicating duelling prowess were at one time much valued in Europe, notably in Germany. Students respected such trophies and poured wine into their wounds to delay the healing and so exaggerate the effect.

Lord Arlington, chamberlain to Charles II, voiced his approval of the damaged male face: 'Scars on the face', he said, 'give a man a fierce and martial air which sets him off to advantage'.

Afghan horsemen, even today, play a game of Buzkashi in which vicious whips are used, often leaving contenders with scars which they treasure for life. In Southern Venezuela, on Feast Days, the Yanomamo Indians enjoy a version of the Scottish sport of tossing the caber – except that they hurl their two-yard-long pieces of wood at their opponent's head. Thereafter, the tops of men's heads are kept carefully shaven to display their impressive scars.

The Punk generation in Britain in the 1970s – females as well as males – pierced their cheeks, noses and ears with safety-pins as part of their anti-authoritarian message. But permanent scars were not the objective. This painful skewering ceased when fake safety-pins became available. The idea was more to shock, and substitute pins and gleaming razor-blades dangling close to the ears looked menacing enough.

Inevitably sex plays its part in facial presentation. Every Tiv woman in Nigeria knows that to be a recognised beauty her face must be intricately incised, oiled and rubbed with henna. To enhance the effect, she often indulges in a kind of temporary tattooing. By pricking her skin with the twig of a special tree she can create white spots, like bleached freckles. Arranged in a formal pattern they can look most effective against her black skin.

Exceptionally, the Tiv engage in modest changes of pattern every ten years or so – but this is more to indicate an individual's generation than to be fashionable. It is, however, an added attraction in the eyes of Tiv women who make it clear that they prefer young, good-looking men bearing new designs. Unfortunately for the men, it is usually the case that the more beautiful the design the greater the pain endured, but this they say is something to be proud of.

'Of course it is painful,' said one of the men when questioned by American anthropologist Paul Bohannan. 'What girl would look at a man if his scars had not cost him pain?'

All in all, the Tiv man aims to please. His skin is his cosmetic currency, and to enhance his sex appeal he will continue to whittle away at it for as long as the flesh will allow. Even scarring with an iron nail is worth a try.

In fact, it looks as though wherever facial markings are sought more for their variety and their sex appeal, than for their value as a social or religious statement, we are back on the same old treadmill and there is the same old restless need for constant change, whatever the price in discomfort and suffering.

6. THE FACE: PERSUASIVE PARTS

The beauty of the face we see springs from the coming together in our minds of all its separate parts. Each part subtly interacts with every other to create a unique, total configuration. Yet quite small changes in any one part can bring about a profound change to the total effect.

DARK LIQUID OR SPARKLING BLUE?

The eyes, considered by many to be the most expressive part of the face, have been a prime target for improvement. In Japan towards the end of the Second World War, it became the fashion for young girls to have their eyes Europeanised to appeal to American soldiers stationed there. Those who did not manage to get a husband in spite of their altered eyes became objects of scorn among their kinsmen. Even today, Japanese moguls and executives elect to have eye surgery to attain what they feel is a more universally successful business image. The flap of eyelid skin, or epicanthic fold, which gives the oriental eye its almond shape is in fact common to all races in the foetal stage in the womb. In Westerners it disappears before birth. Only among Orientals does it remain.

But even the eyes of Westerners become hooded and acquire bags as the years increase. So to maintain their youthful image in an increasingly competitive commercial world – or simply to remain 'young and beautiful' for vanity's sake – they too seek eyelid surgery, blepharoplasty. Pop-star Michael Jackson – as part of his unstoppable campaign to put back the clock and become Peter Pan for ever – had his eyes made rounder in the hope that they would look more 'childlike'. Vidal Sassoon has had his eyes done by Hollywood's Stephen Zax – the boyish look is, after all, part of his trade-mark.

There are hazards. If not done really skilfully, there are often ugly scars and almost always prolonged bruising – which accounts for the periodic disappearance of the fashionably famous to far-away beaches. And the entire operation may, in any case, be a complete waste of time because under-correction can result in no significant difference, whilst over-correction can give a permanently wide-eyed, even desperate look. Some patients find, to their horror, that they are no longer able to close their eyes or even blink, after surgery. Others finish up with eyelids which have become everted, or turned out. And Nature herself can sometimes turn the tables: many people become depressed because they do not like their new eyes after surgery. Some can't even have a good cry about it because they are suffering from a post-operative condition known as 'dry-eye syndrome' – their tear-ducts having dried up. And others have experienced a most unexpected come-uppance – like Robert Mitchum who lost his part in a film because, without the bags under his eyes, he no longer looked rugged enough!

Decorating the eyes is an altogether safer proposition. Whether instinctively or with awareness – or just by the force of fashion and conformity – women have for centuries applied cosmetics to their eyes and eyebrows to accentuate their femininity, and men have plucked their eyebrows. Ancient Egyptians found it useful to use malachite green eye-paste to protect their eyes against light, and this attractive green substance soon became prized for its purely decorative qualities. More recently, in the 1970s, David Vanian of the group The Damned, took to wearing eye make-up with heavy shadow (often purple) around the whole eye both on and off stage. The trade-mark of another group, Kiss involved such spectacular make-up, especially around the eyes, that they boycotted all interviews unless they were wearing their make-up.

Bedouin tribes – both men and women – in the nineteenth century used to stain the whites of their eyes blue with kohl or antimony. They said that this was to sharpen the vision, but the real aim was clearly cosmetic. Antimony sulphide has been used for centuries in the eyes of Egyptians, Romans, Asians and Persians to make them glitter: a dangerous practice since it can result in dried-up tear ducts and even eventually lead to blindness. More recently, since antimony is said to be in short supply, lead sulphide has been taking its place in a product called Surma. Banned in Britain Asian communities are using it when well-meaning friends and relatives bring it back from their travels, as a present. It has been responsible for two deaths in Britain and the applicator rods used to spread it on the eye have caused corneal abrasions.

Antimony sulphide has also been used in kohl for external beautification of the eye – lining the rims, darkening the eyebrow, shadowing the lid – a less harmful pursuit than introducing the substance into the eye itself.

Like the Bedouin, the women of the sixteenth and seventeenth centuries were ready to risk their health. They dropped belladonna into their eyes so that their pupils would dilate and give them a temporarily excited appearance. They felt that this eager, fevered look made them more attractive to the opposite sex. And it probably did, because by dilating the pupils, it darkened their eyes – a strong feminine signal. At the same time, however, it unfortunately robbed the eye of its natural reflex protection against bright light and encouraged the blinding disease of glaucoma. Had these ladies left matters to nature, genuine pleasure and real excitement would probably have enlarged their pupils anyway, and without any artificial help. In both men and women, pupils dilate when looking at pleasant objects, a reaction quite beyond our control. Though we may not be aware of it, when we are gazing, eyeball to eyeball at our loved ones, it is highly likely that we see them through dilated pupils and therefore a larger aperture lens, which as every modern photographer knows, will produce a hazier image. So the beloved's face appears attractively blurred – a neat little trick which Nature plays, perhaps to keep up our numbers.

Jade dealers of the Orient, a thousand years ago, knew all about the give-away signals the eye might make. To conceal their excitement at a particularly fine piece of jewellery, they wore dark spectacles when negotiating prices.

But whether the vision is dimmed with love, or belladonna, the eyes remain an irresistible target for embellishment. Elizabeth Arden's make-up artist Pablo, once declared them 'the only part really worth making up' but then affected some astonishment that women chose to copy and wear his exotic eye designs, some of which took five hours to produce. Spotted eyes had a certain vogue in the late 1960s. Which seems odd really, when so many women go to such lengths to get rid of natural freckles. The choice for dotty eyes was wide – there were polkadot brown or black designs to surround the eyes: alternatively, brightly painted freckles to scatter liberally around the cheekbones. Users were earnestly advised not to wear lipstick at the same time because the look being aimed at was essentially outdoor and 'natural'.

Day-glo paints were a favourite in the 1970s. Multi-coloured polka-dot tears hinting at some kind of technicolour tragedy were strewn across women's faces. David Bowie made a virtue of his differently coloured left and right eyes (the result of a boyhood scrap which permanently dilated one of his pupils). Optical science has also made it possible for anyone by artificial means to have one eye green and another violet. In the seventies, bizarre designs ran riot. One model painted a rainbow around her eyes, reddened her lashes and streaked her hair green. Sales of eye pencils and shadows boomed. In 1981 there was trouble at both Revlon and Maybelline. The latter challenged Revlon's claim that its Formula 2 eyecolour pencil was 'creaseproof'. Revlon were indignant. All we mean, they protested, is that it doesn't collect in the creases of the eyelid in the course of six hours or more. 'No one', they said, 'would expect an eye-shadow to be creaseproof in perpetuity'. The National Advertising Review Board eventually ruled that yes, the advertisement might just have the capacity to be misleading.

The eyelashes' natural function is to protect the eyes. Females are better served than males because female lashes are longer and stronger, though unfortunately, age does tend to wither them. The lashes of neither sex become white with age, but many women have taken to dyeing them simply for novelty. Twiggy's boyfriend Justin de Villeneuve had the bright idea of drawing eyelashes under her eyes. 'He copied them from a doll he had,' said Twiggy. Fashion designer Zandra Rhodes did the same, and coloured hers red. But whatever their colour, long, thick eyelashes have always been considered a desirable attribute and women have always cultivated them. Elizabeth Arden's recommendation in the 1950s was to scrape a razor-blade along black velvet ribbon and then dip a brush, wet with mascara, into the fluff before attacking the lashes to give them a 'velvety texture'. The trick in ancient Rome was to apply powdered lead mixed with water, to give them a dark, luxuriant look. In 1919 in Britain, beauty columnist Celia Cole believed more in 'grow your own'. She recommended a good petroleum jelly at night and saltwater baths in the

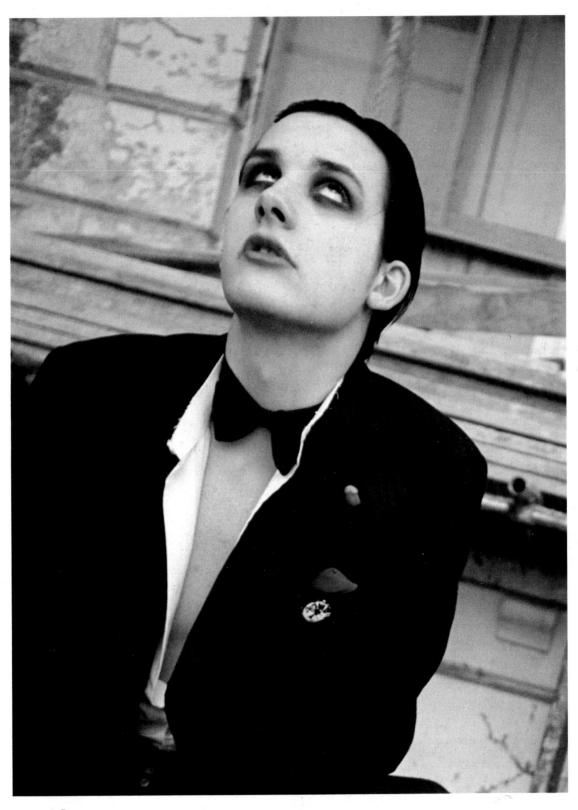

David Vanian of The Damned took to wearing heavy eye make-up both on and off the stage day. At about the same time, a Mrs Pomeroy was employing a different approach: she had a thriving little transplant business in Bond Street, beefing up skimpy eyelashes by removing hairs from the head and sewing them on to the lids. Had they been a little nearer geographically, the Trobrianders of the Western Pacific might have collaborated with Mrs Pomeroy in drumming up business. They regarded the eyelashes as 'the gateways of erotic desire'. At the height of Trobriand passion during love-making, a lover would commonly bite off a portion of his lady's lashes. This playful nibbling was known as 'Mitakuku'.

RAISING AN EYEBROW OR TWO

Eyebrows – those moving goalposts of the beauty business – have been up, down, arched, straight, thick, thin, or even totally banished. In the 1930s everyone wanted arched brows. Because everyone wanted to look like Greta Garbo. Brows were ruthlessly plucked and pencilled to order. Margaret Lockwood shaved hers off altogether and then found they would not grow again – a danger which many other unfortunate women have discovered too late. In Cleopatra's time they substituted their shaved-off brows with painted ones. So did the British in the eighteenth century, but they replaced theirs with artificial eyebrows made of mouse-skin. And this had its own special hazards: without the help of today's Bostiks, there was a tendency for ladies with mobile faces inadvertently to shake off their mouse-skin brows during lively conversation. Some women preferred to keep their own eyebrows, but liked to darken them with the juice of ripe elderberries. Others, unnerved by the elderberry's short season, tortured their brows into shape with primitive tweezers and then blackened them with lead combs, totally ignoring the dangers of the poisonous lead being absorbed into the skin. Sophia Loren – blessed with unusual commonsense in the matter of beautifying – advocates a natural line for the brows. But she confesses freely to using her brows to good purpose. She says she accents them heavily when she wants to intimidate. 'If I want to seem a little more aggressive I use more pencil: when my mood is sweet and gentle, just a feathery brush of pencil does the trick.'

SIGHT FOR SORE EYES

But however useful for beautifying the face or for signalling mood, the eyebrows sometimes have to take second place behind the rake of a spectacle frame. The sad fact is that the majority of people over forty-five begin to have problems focusing because the muscles of the eyes have by this time lost some of their elasticity.

Nowadays, spectacle lenses can correct most faults and weaknesses. It is the choice of frames which preoccupies most spectacle wearers. The idea of different frames for different occasions is catching on. Comedienne Su Pollard, for example, keeps a collection of twenty-two pairs of spectacles, many of them with magnificent 'Dame Edna' frames. For the more affectionate encounter she admits they sometimes cause problems. Head-on collisions with a clashing of frames can be embarrassing. 'Mind you,' she says, 'if I didn't wear them, I wouldn't even know who I was trying to kiss.'

Tinted glasses are not only protective: they add more than a touch of glamour. In the 1960s, the American fashion designer Joan 'Tiger' Morse had a collection of eighty exotic pairs. Spectacular sunglasses of this kind are often worn throughout the waking day – indoors and out – and whatever the weather. But experts in this field – the photobiologists – argue that our eyes need at least one hour's unadulterated light per day if we are not to become irritable and disturbed. Ophthalmologists might disagree.

Some spectacle wearers run into trouble when they want to use eye make-up. How to put on their eye-shadow when they need glasses to see what they are doing? Frames have recently been developed which have hinged lenses designed to flip up independently for just this problem. The left eye can watch what is happening to the right.

Spectacles span all class barriers. Queen Elizabeth wears no-nonsense functional frames. Prince Philip prefers contact lenses. So does Geoffrey Boycott. And so do one and a half million other people in the UK and just under 20 million in the USA. Vanity is not the sole motivation. The absence of frames and freedom from steamed-up, spray-splashed lenses appeals strongly to sportsmen and women. Not even yachtsmen – much plagued with this problem – have so far devised alternative wind-screen-wiper spectacles.

Once upon a time all contact lenses were 'hard'. You kept them in your eyes for a limited amount of time and you had to take them out to clean them, every day. In the early days there were plenty of tales of misadventure with 'hard' lenses. One man left his in for a week. When they were eventually prized away from him, his precious corneas – examined under high magnification – looked, according to the surgeon, 'as pitted and scarred as the moon's surface'.

Nowadays you can buy either 'hard' or 'soft' lenses. 'Hard' lenses are now made which are 'gas permeable'. They can be left in for seven days at a stretch and the eye will receive adequate oxygen. But all contact lenses demand the strictest discipline from the user. If those lenses intended for use for only a limited time during the day are left in for longer, they bring about oxygen starvation. This causes the cornea to swell, which may not be immediately apparent. Even if the forgetful wearer eventually remembers to remove them before becoming uncomfortable, he/she may well find, two or three hours afterwards, that there is considerable pain – and often hazy vision caused by conjunctival infection. It is very worrying when it happens and frightened users have often required to be sedated – sometimes for as long as two days after the trauma.

There are plenty of other hazards. Stories of lost lenses are legion. Relaxing in chair or sofa it is all too easy for the unwary to nod off leaving the lens to slip upwards under the upper lid and get stuck. Opticians are often called out to lend a hand in recovery, usually after distraught users have spent hours searching carpets and scouring upholstery for these precious items.

It is hard luck if you opt to wear contact lenses and then turn out to be allergic to your own tears. Meticulous lens-cleaning then becomes absolutely crucial. But even then, sensitivity to the chemical solutions used to clean and disinfect and store lenses remains a common problem, as well as being an expensive one. Users in this sort of difficulty are well advised to consult a practitioner. The cure may be a different wetting solution which may in fact consist of nothing more than 99.9% water and 0.1% salt, but which can be expensive.

But in spite of all the problems, the popularity of contact lenses seems undiminished. Manufacturers are prospering in a growing market and are now producing lenses which are ever more sophisticated. Some soft lenses are now being advertised as suitable for 'extended wear' – theoretically they can be left in for a month without cleaning. But most opticians are wary of these claims. The chances of infection are much lessened by taking the trouble to clean them once a week, rather than once a month.

A new idea has come recently from Scandinavia: lenses which are disposable – designed to be worn for a fortnight and then thrown away. But this has generated new problems for men and women who cannot resist the temptation to make them last longer.

There are additional hazards for those who normally use cosmetics. These wearers of contact lenses should steer clear of glittering eye gels, fibrous mascaras and loose powder eye-shadows – particles can all too easily escape into the eyes and damage or irritate them. Special hypo-allergenic eye-shadow creams have now been created to overcome this difficulty.

A new idea, fresh on the fashion scene, is the use of contact lenses which have been decorated in some way. Mystique have developed a clear contact lens with coloured flecks to blend with the natural colour of the iris. The TV actress Sally Whittaker treated herself to a green-tinted pair. They turned to be a mistake. 'I looked like a cat,' she said. And one should beware of being captivated by a pair of sparkling eyes – be they blue, green or brown. Not everyone may be honest enough to allow the coloured scales to drop from their eyes . . . at least right away. Fashion may well overtake this hazard. Very soon, those who can afford them may be equipping themselves with an arsenal of coloured lenses to choose from, according to the colour of a dress or sweater, or even the mood of the day. Already there are quite a few wearers of coloured contact lenses who don't need glasses at all.

More exotic still – though perhaps a touch expensive at £650 a pair – are the new clear lenses with what one might describe as a little extra on the side. The lenses are decorated peripherally with, as you wish, 'a heart, or even a country scene'. How quaint to gaze into one's loved-one's eyes and at the same time be able to view their miniature Turners or Constables, or may be a coded message of love?

THE PERFECT MOUTH

As expressive and vital as the eyes, the mouth is perhaps the must erotic organ of the face. When film-star Clara Bow in the late 1920s translated her surname to her lips, women everywhere wanted an upper lip with a cupid's bow, just like hers. Very soon cosmetic houses were selling the 'Q' BO Lip Mask, to stencil in your own lips as adroitly as tracing a Laura Ashley rose on to an ageing chest-of-drawers. Just place the shield over the lips, said the makers, trace in the bow and 'you will have a perfect mouth'. What they really meant was you could achieve the mouth that was then in fashion.

When considered in proportion to the size of the face, female lips are slightly bigger than those of the male. Hence the urge, albeit often unconscious, to make them even more conspicuous to stress femininity. Enlarging their outline and exaggerating their colour are two obvious ways of doing this. And this has led women – and sometimes men too – to experiment with pigments and dyes of every description, and even to tattooing their lips. In Japan, the hairy Ainu women used to exaggerate their mouths by tattooing a larger mouth around the real one. Yanomamo women opted for decoration rather than size and demonstrated their femininity even more directly: at their first menstruation they tattooed their upper lip with the sickle moon.

But it is not always appropriate simply to enlarge the lips and intensify their colour. Subtler considerations must be taken into account – like the 'simultaneous contrast' effect of skin colour against lips and lips against teeth. Sophia Loren's advice for those whose maturing teeth have yellow tones is to avoid the red/purple ranges of lipsticks and go for corals and orange/reds.

During the cosmetic shortages of the Second World War, lipstick was the item of make-up women said they missed most. They had a greater psychological dependence on it than on any other cosmetic. Service personnel and nurses, transported overseas and restricted to a very few personal possessions, invariably included a lipstick.

In America, in 1924, J. H. Collins, a journalist on *The Saturday Evening Post*, started a minor scare: he reckoned that 50 million American women were being kissed every day by, at least, 50 million American men. 'Is there a danger', he asked, 'that the men will be poisoned?' It was enough to stimulate the New York Board of Health into collecting and analysing lipstick samples which, happily, turned out to be harmless. The same cannot be said of the poisonous red fucus – a lethal dye containing mercuric sulphide – which Elizabethan ladies used for colouring their lips. Of course the possible toxicity factor in lipsticks is very important: the lips are especially sensitive and inevitably a great deal of lipstick is ingested. The firm of Fabergé once attempted to turn the 'eating' of lipstick into a positive delight: they introduced caramel-flavoured lipstick, followed by 'Graype' and 'Pistachio'. Cutex, too, tried to sweeten the lips to make them 'tawny, toasty, terrific'. But the idea did not catch on.

In late Victorian polite society, the rule was that married ladies could lightly rouge their cheeks to counter the 'green sickness'. But they must never colour their lips. These could be 'tinted only with the hues of health' according to one authoritative text. When dry, however, they might possibly be allowed a little cold cream. And no doubt many women were glad of this concession since it was common practice to bite the lips hard and so encourage colour, before approaching a social gathering in a drawing room.

In ancient folk legends there are many references to the 'all-consuming fiery mouth' and these tales have inevitably sparked off much psycho-analytic speculation about deeper significances. Certainly the mouth has powerful unconscious associations – which is why its decoration has always been so widely practised among tribal societies. It has, for example, manifested itself in folk tales as the 'vagina-dentata', an orifice with teeth, ready to bite off any venturesome organs of male sexuality. Physiognomists, philosophers and poets are more gently disposed to the mouth and lips. In his *Moral Thoughts*, Tommaseo thought the mouth was 'the repository of the soul'. J. C. Lavater, the most impressive and widely-quoted physiognomist of all time described it as, 'so sacred to me that I scarcely dare speak of it. It is eloquent even in its silence.'

But the precise symbolism underlying the more exotic alterations of the mouth employed by non-Western peoples, is sometimes difficult to decide. Whether a particular decoration has its roots in old legends, whether it has some special significance at a sub-conscious level, or whether it is simply indicating some sort of tribal affiliation or rite of passage, is often hard to distinguish.

In Northern Cameroon, for example, young women have their lips pierced at adolescence. At the same time, they are talked to about the 'facts of life' or as they prefer to put it, further enlightened about the 'things of women'. The details of this special inside information for women are said to have been passed down by ancestors who first heard about them from a frog. So it is natural enough that their lip ornaments have evolved with a frog-like look.

In Brazil, among the Suya community a youth has his lips pierced when he leaves 'the world of women' and enters into the men's house. Once here, he contemplates marriage and, whilst waiting, his companions insert lip discs of increasing size into his lower lip. As a mature man he will rarely remove them – perhaps only to wash – but on feast days he rejoices by draping his discs with tassels and other eye-catching decorations.

Young Botocudo girls in another part of Brazil work hard at achieving a grotesque spoon-bill lip. The enormous discs they insert in their mouths, sometimes as much as thirty inches around, might be expected to inhibit speech, and Dr David Livingstone seems to have found this to be the case in Africa, where he reported that women wearing their labrets were 'to all practical purposes, dumb'. These discs, or labrets, which are sometimes worn in pairs in both upper and lower lips by African people undoubtedly do

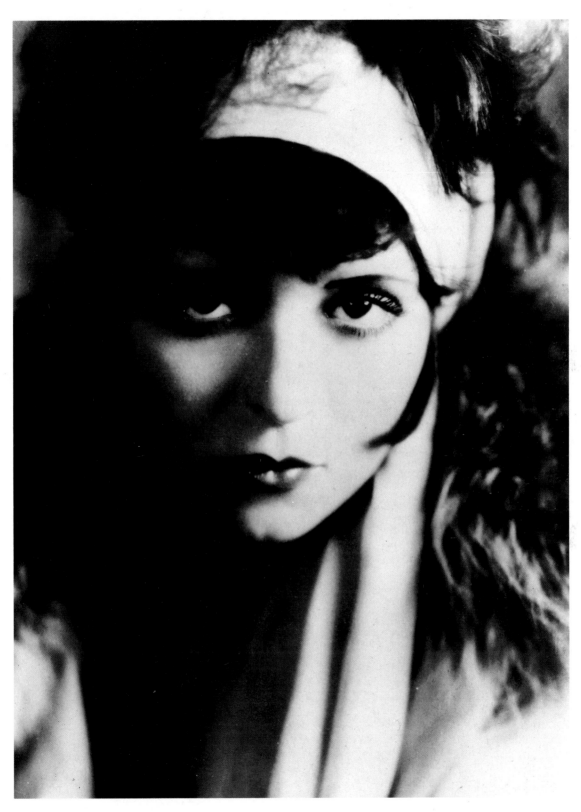

Clara Bow, whose perfectly formed 'Cupid's bow' lips set a whole fashion for the
1920s

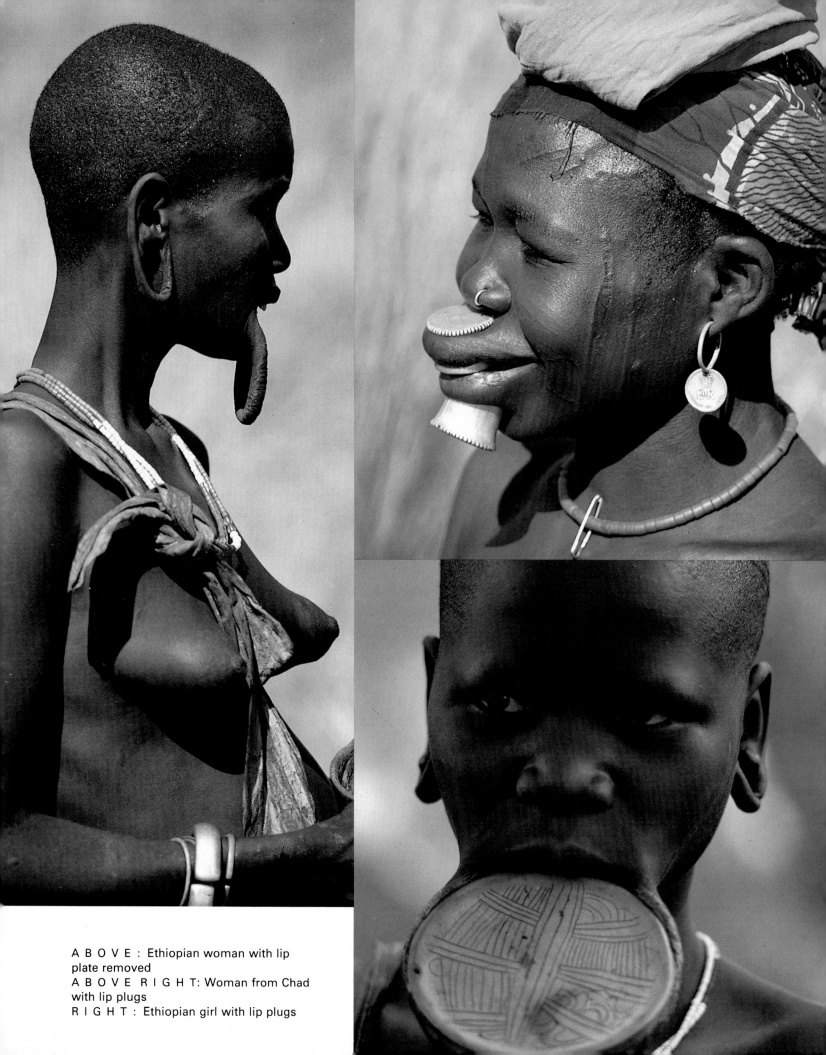

A B O V E : Ethiopian woman with lip
plate removed
A B O V E   R I G H T: Woman from Chad
with lip plugs
R I G H T : Ethiopian girl with lip plugs

make their speech much more difficult, sometimes impossible; they tend to rattle together, as their owners give voice. Yet the experience of others has been different. When the Rock star, Sting went to Brazil in 1988 to meet Raoni, the 'Stone Age Chief', Raoni spoke quite clearly despite the enormous plate in his lip.

Lip discs are sometimes used as status symbols. The Thlinkits of NW Canada grade theirs according to the rank of the wearer: large bone ones for homely folk and silver ones for the more elevated. The Dessin women of West Africa, on the other hand, find lip plugs and tusks more to their taste.

In the West cosmetic surgery is frequently used to change the mouth to conform to current notions of beauty. For example, surgeons can help us to have a V-shaped piece removed from the centre line and the edges joined together again, should we feel orally overendowed; or if too small, to have an incision made in the centre with flesh grafted between the exposed edges. Much more popular are the silicone substances which can be injected for dealing with those fine, give-away lines which develop and cluster above the mouth. Starved and chilly-looking lips may be tattooed to give them a permanent warmth. Even tongues can be tattooed if you have a taste for it – though tattoo-enthusiasts themselves admit that it's excruciatingly painful.

Paradoxically, lip discs among the Ubangi of Africa were not originally used to make the womenfolk attractive: quite the reverse – they were to make them as repulsive as possible to slave traders. Occasionally too, women were 'disfigured' in this way to dampen down tribal jealousies. But then, the bizarre, fascinating look of the stretched lip began to attract more and more attention – and, instead of putting people off, curiosity was aroused, and then interest in the technique, then admiration. After that it was but a short step to considering the projecting lip beautiful. And only a matter of time before lips were being punished into sizes big enough to hold a canister of motion picture film – a feat achieved by one African lady, in 1938. The can, so proudly displayed, was big enough to hold 400 feet of film. And the lady's lip was so elastic that, when pulled, it snapped back 'like a rubber band'.

BARING ONE'S TEETH

However perfect one's physical features, a smile which reveals nasty teeth will ruin a face. Long before she became famous, Emma, Lady Hamilton, was once on the point of selling her fine young teeth to a vain old woman. Happily, she changed her mind. But many a young servant girl in the eighteenth century took the money and went ahead with premature extractions. The reasoning was simple. Withdraw the bad old teeth of the rich and immediately replace them with good ones, newly-extracted, from the poor . . . and then hope for the best. The idea was two hundred years before its time, and it was not a success. Stability of the newly-planted tooth was poor and infection frequently arose

O P P O S I T E : In many societies extending and plugging the lips have been revered methods of beautification between implant and natural tissue. Two or three months' use at the most was all that could be expected from an implant and then only from an exceptionally good – or lucky – strike. But this did not deter resolute old women in search of a born-again smile. So countless numbers of bright young teeth were sacrificed needlessly.

Similarly in the north of England at the turn of this century a father's wedding present to his daughter was quite often the money to have all her teeth removed and false ones provided. The idea of this dental dowry was that it would save trouble and expense for bride and groom in years to come.

Nowadays, cosmetic dentistry offers many alternatives for the rehabilitation of stained and much-filled teeth. A failing tooth can be filed down to a post and a 'cap' cemented over it. If the tooth is already non-vital all is not lost. The tooth can be made sterile and a metal post inserted into the root as an anchoring post.

When teeth are unhappily lost for ever there are, of course, removable dentures. Or in the case of just one or two missing teeth, a bridge can be fitted. Old-style bridges had false teeth attached to crowns which were fitted to filed-down teeth on either side of the gap. New-style bridges still require the support teeth on either side but, instead of being filed down, they are grooved to receive a false tooth with metal wings which slot into the grooves. Also bridges can now be etched to the adjacent teeth by means of wings attached to the pontic which spans the space to be filled – altogether less traumatic solutions than the sacrificial filing down of perfectly good teeth.

Film stars – with close-up smiles to consider – have in the past endured such filing simply to provide themselves with a set of better-looking capped teeth. Good, serviceable teeth were not enough – they had to look white, regular and perfect. Sometimes, instead of drastic filing, stars used temporary veneers to cover up stained teeth, but these had to be removed after each day's filming.

Now, stained and much-filled teeth can be more permanently transformed by etching them with acid and then bonding to them perfectly-fitting opaque veneers (rather like false finger-nails). If the veneers themselves should eventually discolour, the treatment can be successfully repeated using new veneers. This is now a well-proven, successful technique and one which has changed the whole face of dentistry in the past few years.

And there is more. If a tooth should require radical re-shaping, then tooth-coloured composite material can be sculpted and bonded to it to produce much the same effect as a veneer. Porcelain – though more expensive – can also be shaped and bonded in this way. And porcelain is much more versatile. Since it is blessed with greater inherent strength, it can be used to extend a tooth beyond its natural edge – and the tooth will still be game for biting an apple. That same tooth can also be 'distressed' with artificial cracks and shadings so that it will not look so suspiciously perfect.

Bleaching is another newly-developed technique for brightening up dingy teeth. For this, a rubber dam is placed around the area to be treated and a chemical solution – usually a strong oxidising agent – is applied and then exposed to heat and light. Even non-vital teeth can be given a cosmetic lift by injecting the bleaching solution into the tooth.

As for those old-fashioned 'St Trinian's' braces, worn so patiently and for so long by youngsters with crowded teeth – an orthodontist from Beverly Hills, California, has done away with them once and for all. Craven Kurtz believes that teeth should be straightened. But, he says, 'no-one wants a scrap-metal smile' during the straightening period. So he has invented invisible braces which fit behind the teeth instead of in front of them. Undetected but effective, they are already being worn by 20,000 American men and women, and of course children.

Much greater advances are in prospect. At a meeting of the British Association in Belfast, in 1987, Professor Mark Ferguson, head of the Department of Cell and Structural Biology at Manchester University, said that he believes it should be possible to vaccinate against tooth decay in the future. When that day comes, toothpastes and toothbrushes will become a thing of the past. Meanwhile though, if extraction is unavoidable, then one consolation is the possibility of dentures made from real human dental enamel which has been produced synthetically by genetic engineering. Even more startling is Professor Ferguson's further prediction that within the next 100 years, it should be possible to transplant cells from human embryos into adults, there to grow and form replacement teeth.

Erling Johannsen, Dean of Dentistry at Tufts University, Boston, has a simpler solution. He believes he has discovered a calcium-phosphate mouthwash that will reach the parts even dental floss cannot explore and which will, at the same time, strengthen and repair both tooth and root. But he puts in a good word for old-fashioned chewing-gum too – providing it is unsweetened. Chewing-gum lowers the pH of the area: it encourages us to salivate and saliva washes off the acids which attack the surface of the tooth.

Nothing like this was available for men and women in past centuries. Their teeth were responsible for more than their smile – they could alter their lifestyle. Because of their poor teeth, eighteenth-century wits learned to cultivate a dry, ironic manner and they avoided smiling. Even that master of the nineteenth-century *bon mot*, Oscar Wilde, was described as looking furtive when he was telling his jokes: he always put his hand in front of his mouth to conceal his poor teeth.

His Victorian contemporaries often chose to eat in their bedrooms before dinner to safeguard themselves against disasters at table. And Disraeli could not resist a sly dig at Palmerston: if he were not so hesitant in his speech, he said, his teeth would almost certainly fall out. For politicians poor teeth were a great drawback. George Washington suffered dreadfully with dentures carved out of ivory – possibly with a few human teeth too – though not, as rumour had it, made from wood or from elk teeth. There was little

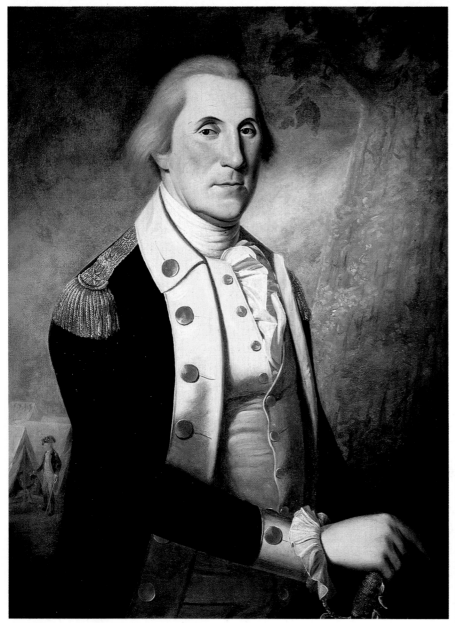

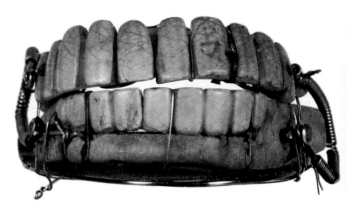

George Washington's false teeth were hinged with wire, which explains why he avoided public speaking in later life

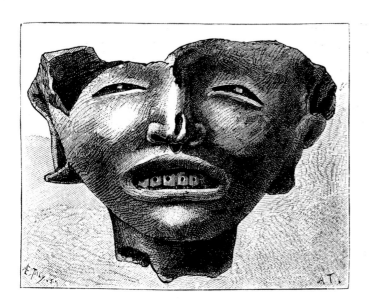

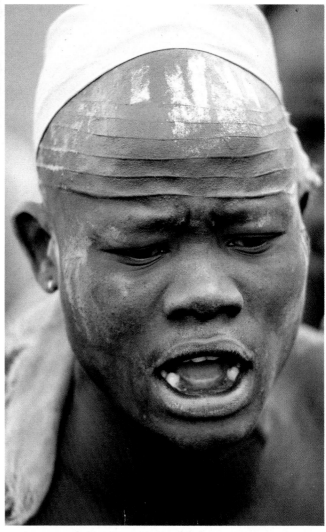

prosthetic dentistry available in his day, and he had to struggle with partial dentures held together with wire. One of his sets was made up of no less than five separate parts held together by gold ligatures. Eventually he became reluctant to speak in public because his false teeth made his voice sound 'hollow and indistinct'. At about the same time in Paris, people sometimes pierced their gums so that a row of teeth fitted with two hooks could be suspended from them; they were known as 'floating teeth'.

By the 1880s it was possible to have a full set of dental plates but still no crowns or bridges. Yet the idea of bridging was an old one. It had clearly occurred to the ancient Greeks who bound their loose teeth with gold wire and tied artificial ones to neighbouring teeth with ligatures. And a bridging appliance was successfully produced by the Etruscans for supporting a replacement for a missing tooth. There was in fact little real progress in restorative dentistry right up to the middle of the nineteenth century.

During Elizabeth's I reign poor diet and lack of knowledge about teeth rapidly annihilated the teeth of even the most aristocratic of ladies. The Sovereign herself possessed yellowed, broken teeth which were irregular and – in later years – quite black. Her use of the popular lead-based ceruse as a cosmetic may have been partially responsible. As John Bulwer, in his *Anthropometamorphosis* of 1650 pointed out, there was a venomous quality in this paint 'which wrinkleth the face before its time . . . it dims the eyes and blacks the teeth'.

It was not that fashionable ladies ignored their teeth; on the contrary, they often made desperate attempts to improve them. One writer in 1773 declared that scrubbing the teeth with gunpowder would give them 'an inconceivable whiteness'. Soon after that, soot was being strongly recommended.

But not all ladies, or gentlemen, want white teeth. Well into the nineteenth century, it was the custom for Japanese prostitutes to paint their faces white and their teeth black. Among some Indonesian tribes teeth have been artificially blackened in an effort to make the mouth appear larger. These Indonesians were heard to refer scornfully to European teeth as being 'like the teeth of a dog'.

In order to enhance their masculinity Boloki men chisel the upper incisors to V-shaped points. Men from the Nicobar Islands in the Indian Ocean seem even more powerfully influenced by their teeth when it comes to masculinity. They would never dream of making sexual advances unless their teeth had been blackened first.

In the Philippines, Bagobo girls used to sharpen their teeth to a point and then blacken them. Malayan girls – blessed with naturally good teeth – used to file them in the interests of beauty. For the Sart women of Russian Turkestan, the spaces left when they lost a tooth or two were considered particularly ugly. Their solution was to paint all the remaining teeth black to hide the gaps.

Masai women in East Africa, like the Kikuyus, filed a triangular notch in their two upper

OPPOSITE : A fashion of piercing teeth appears to have existed in Ancient Mexico, while the Dinka of Southern Sudan knock out their front teeth to improve their looks and as a safety precaution against lockjaw.

incisors. The Masai found this was really quite useful: they acquired the art of spitting through the gap, a mark of great respect and friendship.

Aborigine girls in Australia favoured the knocking out of a front tooth. Baluba women of the Congo went one – or rather three – better; they knocked out the four front incisors and then had the remainder of their teeth filed to sharp points.

Melanesian women, like many other Orientals and South Asians, content themselves with chewing Areca nut, betel, pepper leaf and lime to redden their mouth. This builds up the very desirable attribute of a substantial black incrustation on the teeth. Many Asian men like it. They say that the gummy, babylike look it gives to their women makes them appear even more pleasingly subordinate.

At first sight these may seem very curious practices. But there have been similarly eccentric fashions in the West, such as using red-tinted toothpaste to make the teeth flash whiter against the strong, bright red of the gums. Or decorating a chosen tooth with a jewel. Or having a front tooth filled with gold. Gold is undoubtedly a stable substance for fillings – but dentists have reported requests for an individual's initials, or those of his favourite pop-star, to be worked in gold on the very visible front teeth. On the whole though, the Western ideal has always been to strive for a full set of pleasingly white teeth against healthily pink gums.

But we do seem to have this habit of changing our minds about perfection – especially when we have achieved it, or nearly achieved it. Which raises the question – supposing Professor Ferguson's best hopes are realised and science does eventually succeed in conquering decay, giving us all the option of a lifetime of perfect white teeth: how long before we become bored with them?

After all, if we find it hard to resist drawing pictures on our contact lenses, who knows what we might get up to once we have mastered our teeth?

A CLOSE SHAVE?

Of the hair that surrounds the mouth, even the free-thinking lesbian author Wendy Chapkis has found herself having to do some hard thinking. On the one hand, her feminist sensibilities are in revolt at bowing to the conventions about facial hair and beauty. Yet she has to confess that facial hair makes a woman feel ugly.

'Men have facial hair; women do not,' is a sentiment unlikely to change.

Nowadays, women attend to unwanted hair with tweezers, or razors, experiment with depilatory creams and pads, or seek the help of an electrolysist. Or more recently they can sugar their unwanted hair away. Tunisian Zahra Benamore uses a 'thick honey-like preparation based on sugar and containing only natural substances'. She is now in business with 120 trained practitioners operating in Britain. Sugaring is an art practised by

Arabian women for centuries, she says. In North Africa, girls are sugared from top to toe before their wedding because hair is considered unclean on a woman.

Electrolysis, pioneered in the 1940s, is perhaps a better-known method of permanent hair removal. The work is skilled, entailing the introduction of a fine needle probe through which a small electric current passes into the tiny root of the hair. It is not without its discomforts and dangers. The operator needs a delicate touch to know when she has reached the base of each follicle. If she misses the root, the hair will grow again. Excessive use of current – especially in sensitive areas such as above the eyes – causes skin damage. According to one report 'scarring may occur, infection can follow and regrowth rates, depending on the skill of the operator, can be as high as 50%'. In any case, the client's will to succeed is crucial. She must, for example, be prepared to allow the offending hairs to grow for a while and become conspicuously visible before treatment can take place. But given persistence and a carefully chosen practitioner, women can nowadays be safely rid of the burden of unwanted facial hair. The British Association of Electrolysists keeps a register of qualified, practising members.

In the eighteenth century the Duke of Newcastle settled £400 a year on the French barber who shaved the upper lip of the Duchess. At that time too, home-made depilatory creams were popular. One recipe required the shells of 52 eggs. Another recommended cat's hard, dry dung which had to be beaten to a powder and then mixed with strong vinegar. For a long period during the Middle Ages, it was not just the hair on the upper lip which was held to be superfluous – forehead hairlines were cropped as well. The babylike look of a tall, high brow was so desirable that women were prepared to wind bandages impregnated with vinegar and cat's dung around their heads in the hope that hair would stop growing. And optimistic mothers conscientiously rubbed walnut oil over children's foreheads to prevent further growth. Quick-lime was another favourite 'remover' though often enough it burned away the skin as well as the hair.

In modern times women whose brows are considered too low for beauty sometimes have them raised. Max Factor plucked the hairline of brunette Rita Cansino to give her a more attractive, high forehead. Then he dyed her hair red. And then she became Rita Hayworth.

Hormones play a crucial part in hair growth. Glandular changes increase the likelihood of upper-lip growth after the menopause. Some contraceptive pills too have encouraged unwelcome hair growth in young women, especially around the nipples. But now there is a further danger. Working with a research team at Cambridge University, Professor Ivor Mills, an endocrinologist, has found that an increasing number of women are suffering from 'stress disease' and are already displaying alarming symptoms of associated hormonal changes such as loss of fertility, growth of facial hair, hair on the abdomen and breasts and even, in some cases, signs that they are beginning to go thin on top. His research team has warned that too many women are taking on more work than they can cope with, full-time jobs, home, children; hence the stress. The delicate 'endocrine orchestra', as the scientist Hoskins once called it, seems in danger of becoming grossly out of tune.

Of course, fads and fancies among women as to whether to wear 'masculine' clothes are simply matters of taste; women can take them or leave them to suit themselves. But one thing is clear: no woman wants to wake up in the morning and be confronted in her mirror with something that looks like the Laughing Cavalier in a nightie. Trousers, big shoulders, collars and ties for women may come and go – facial hair, never. In this one area, at least, women have never had aspirations to look like men. There have been, however, one or two curious exceptions. Goddess figures were often shown bearded and this was held to give them greater importance and significance. Queen Matshrtpdont of ancient Egypt, just like the Pharaohs, wore a ceremonial beard to mark her authority and majesty. Luckily for her, it was a false one, appropriately jewelled and gilded.

Attitudes to men's facial hair have been much less consistent. Men themselves seem to like it but they are not always sure about flaunting it. Chopin's bizarre compromise was to shave only one side of his face: 'I always sit with my right cheek to the audience,' he said.

An old Maori proverb says, 'There is no woman for a hairy man'. But in ancient Babylon a beard was considered a sign of virility and strength. In Greece, Diogenes used to taunt clean-shaven men with the cry: 'What sex are you?'

Wearing a beard in ancient Egypt was once the special privilege of rulers. The upper classes were also allowed to wear them, usually artificial ones, carefully graded in size to indicate the owner's rank and authority. But twentieth-century television producers have recently turned this idea about beards giving authority, completely on its head. Just the reverse, they say. 'Beards lack authority, especially on the small screen.' They sometimes decline to use interviewees who have facial hair. But could it be that beards are so powerfully intimidating and so very full of authority that TV producers prefer to remain unthreatened by them? Is this a minor manifestation of 'pogonophobia', the medical term for terror of beards?

Pop musicians have experimented with all manner of whiskers, and styles of music seem to have found an echo in facial hair styles: sideburns for the Rockabillies; goatees for the folk and jazz brigade; dramatic Zapata moustaches to go with the psychedelic sound.

Most men possessing beards have, by and large, cosseted them. Like the Assyrians they have oiled, scented, curled them – even sprinkled them with gold dust. Sir Thomas More demonstrated his affection for his beard when, at the execution block, he moved it gently to one side 'my beard has not been guilty of treason'.

At other times beards have been out of favour. Around 1910 in Britain, and in the inter-war years, all but older men were clean-shaven. The only other exceptions were the military. Moustaches were allowed in the Army, and full beards for men in the Navy. Desmond Morris says that a man shaving off his beard is declaring that he is prepared to be friendly and ready to stifle his ancient, aggressive urges. As for the significance of that compromise the moustache – the chin can no doubt be shaved to demonstrate friendliness, but it might be as well to leave a reminder of fighting potential on the upper lip. Cash Cooper has made sure of this by tattooing an extra moustache on himself beneath his natural one. In fact he did it as a competition entry – and maybe for publicity. His motto was, 'In God we trust: all others pay Cash.' Victorian gentlemen often exploited their 'fighting potential' by waxing their moustaches to points as fine as those on the head of a twentieth-century Punk. In America moustache-waxing enjoyed a revival in the late Fifties.

In the last decade, however, in New York and San Francisco, and in London, moustaches suddenly acquired a new significance when they came to be worn as a gay 'come hither' signal. Heterosexuals rapidly shaved theirs off.

But there is one cardinal difference between male and female attitudes to hairiness which is that for women, removal must be a dark secret. Little is ever volunteered about consultations with electrolysists. This is one of the few feminine preoccupations which remains intact and unspoken.

Men, on the other hand, sustain and enhance their masculine image by making completely public their need to shave. Removing hair could be a painful business though. Julius Caesar, like the Sumerians, had his facial hair plucked out with tweezers – and so did Beau Brumell. It was no secret. So however beardless they appeared in public, everyone knew they were proper, thoroughly hairy men underneath.

The 'New Man' of the 1980s may have his skin softened by creams; he may attempt a closer shave with the 'double-concave-headed millimetre foil-thin shavers' which have replaced the old cut-throat; he may dry-shave with an electric shaver, reassuringly backed up with a skin soother. But whatever the type of shave, and whatever the soother used, we all know that within twenty-four hours that familiar stubborn blue shadow will be creeping back. In the late 1970s a glimpse of this masculine growth suddenly became all the rage. Even the fresh-faced Cliff Richard began to appear with five o'clock shadow. And nowadays, what better than deliberately to cultivate the fashionable 'designer stubble'? You can buy a shaver head which leaves exactly ⅛″ all round – or even more, if you wish.

Pop-star George Michael regularly appears with substantial bristles springing out through his make-up, virile and ready to grate on a willing female cheek. Women cannot fail to be roused by such clear-cut and visible emphasis on this major difference between the sexes. For there is no mistaking the message. Even more strongly accented by designer stubble than through beard or moustache, the proposition is clear – within every smooth-cheeked man there's a very potent male bursting to get out.

NOSE JOBS

Behind his back, his soldiers called him 'Nosy'. But the Duke of Wellington regarded his high, arched nose as his most distinguished feature and the one which especially enhanced his commanding presence. Napoleon, too, admired and placed much reliance on men with strong noses. 'Give me a man with a good allowance of nose,' he said. But that was before Waterloo.

We all have very clear ideas about the implications of different nasal shapes for character and personality and, particularly, sexuality. We sense that big, arched noses are strong and masculine. Small, concave noses are babylike and very feminine. And these impressions are, in fact, based on differences between males and females which are real enough: male noses are often bigger and more convex than female noses.

The Romans firmly believed that the length of a man's nose was an indication of virility. Even these days, remarks about a man's 'Roman Nose' are usually taken as a compliment. Desmond Morris's explanation for this is that the male has only two substantial appendages springing from the centre-line of his body, and the sizes of these two have become linked in the unconscious. The bigger the nose, the greater the masculine endowment.

Morris carries the analogy further. According to him, sexual arousal increases the size of the male nose – at least temporarily; at moments of high passion it becomes engorged with blood and the springy tissue making up much of the side walls of the nose demonstrates an unexpected erectile potential. And, he asserts, it becomes hotter too. One conscientious researcher, though perhaps understandably distracted, has evidently proved this to be true by comparing the temperature of a nose going about its everyday business and a nose in the emotional throes of love-making.

Surprising then, that men with large noses have ever been prepared to reduce them – unless perhaps they are finding more favour by presenting today's feminist women with a less challenging phallic symbol. Simple aesthetic considerations too may underlie the desire for change. Ambitions for elegance rather than more macho preoccupations may have motivated the pop singer Tom Jones and Wham's Andrew Ridgeley who have both had their sizeable noses neatly tailored.

For women, the small nose is a highly desirable attribute. The secret lies in its impression of youth. The faces of babies happen to be disproportionately short from eyes to nostrils, leaving room for only a tiny smudge of a nose. And it is this endearing button-nose of the baby which is said to encourage in adults such a feeling of protectiveness. This, combined with the notion that what is young must also be healthy, and what is healthy must also be beautiful, makes the small nose attractively appealing.

Television personalities – Cilla Black and Marti Cane – make no secret of their nose bobs. Barbara Goalen, 'Queen of the Mannequins' in the 1950s and a strong believer in tidying things up at the edges, had her nose bobbed to make her face more beautiful.

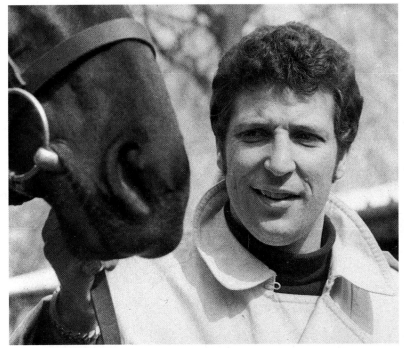

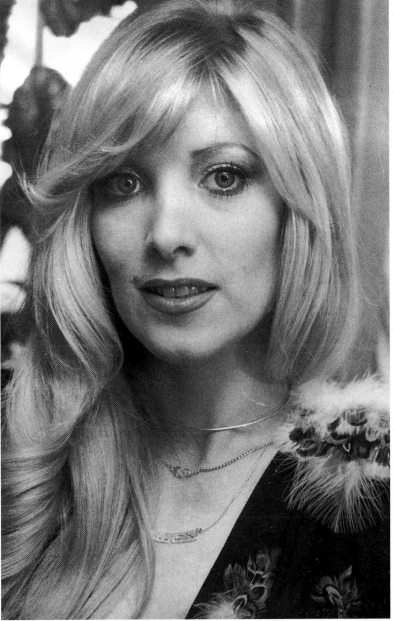

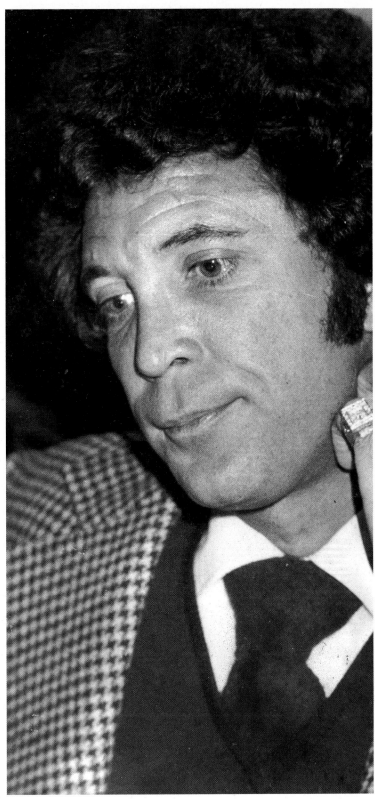

Tom Jones before and after nose reduction

Lynsey de Paul: 'A nose job is never a thing to be undertaken lightly'

Earlier this century, the advice to women who felt their nose was too broad was to try out a 'nasal clamp' – a contraption which was fastened over the ears with an elastic band and then adjusted over the nose with small screws. *Vogue* was full of encouragement, especially since the clamp was quite safe and – they reassured – could be relied upon to 'gently shape the sides of the nose without impeding the breathing'. A Seventies' model, Lauren Hutton, confessed to a much less complicated method: she had used a clothes-peg to pinch and point up the offending tip of her nose.

Nowadays, and significantly perhaps in a feminist climate when women are more than ever pleasing themselves about their appearance, an increasing number of successful stars are resisting interference with their 'strong' noses. Sophia Loren, for example, sincerely believes that if you shorten a nose, the face loses its 'special strength and beauty'. Meryl Streep and Barbra Streisand too have determinedly hung on to their distinctive noses. What is there to be gained by standardisation? Personality, individuality, not conformity, is the cry.

Yet the nose is such a tempting target for alteration. And alteration can make such a profound difference to the overall appearance of the face. Leonardo da Vinci was convinced that it was the nose above all else that established the psychological character of the face. Pascal believed that if Cleopatra had had a different nose 'the whole face of the earth would have been changed'. Dürer demonstrated, in his drawings, what strange and remarkable alterations may be brought about by simply altering the size of the nose. More recently, a new device designed to help the police identify criminals (The Liggett Facial Synthesiser) allows facial outlines and features to be altered in size and position on a TV screen. This has clearly demonstrated that the slightest alteration in nose size can dramatically change facial appearance.

For purely practical reasons too, the nose is an ideal structure for re-vamping. One of the big attractions of this 'rhinoplasty' is that surgery can almost always be undertaken from within the nostrils so that any scars remain unseen. Cartilage – the stuff that much of the hard structure of the nose is made up of – can be attacked from the inside with a small bayonet saw and removed without trace.

But, as with any cosmetic surgery, much can go wrong, and especially if the credentials of the surgeon are at all in doubt. Many unsuspecting patients have suffered at the hands of unscrupulous practitioners. Recently one woman had a nose-bob during which too much bone was removed. The nose drooped, she was unable to breathe through it, and she could no longer swallow.

Even an innocent post-operative sneeze can sometimes throw nasal stitches and packing into disorder, and necessitate a second operation.

Sometimes too, modest initial success can lead to over-ambition and disaster. The singer, Lynsey de Paul suffered from a large nose and large nostrils. Her nose, she said,

OPPOSITE : Sophia Loren believes that if you shorten a nose the face loses its 'special strength and beauty'

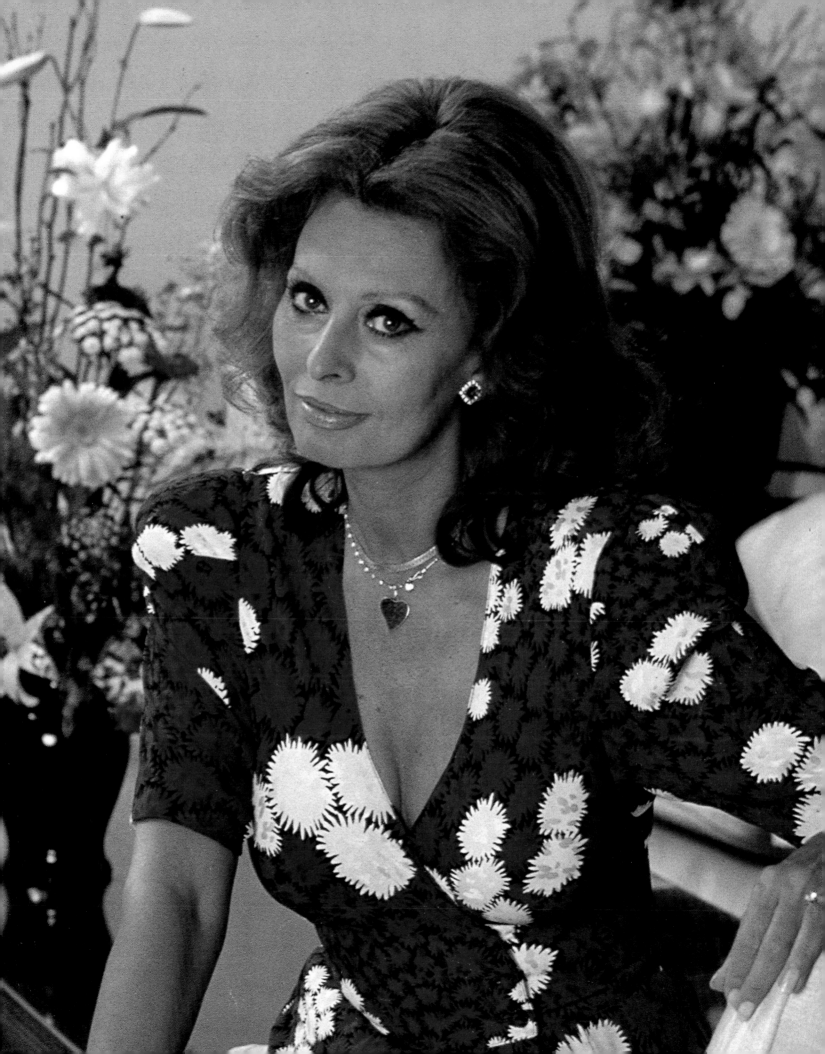

'was so big I could put my two index fingers up it simultaneously without discomfort. It was terrible. It's no laughing matter, a big nose.' She had her first nose-bob at the age of seventeen. The success of this led her to have another operation – one which she admits was not, strictly speaking, necessary. And it went sadly wrong. In an interview describing her second operation Miss de Paul grimly recounted 'the pain', 'the bone grafts', and 'the splinters taken from my ribs'. 'Now I realise that a nose job is never a thing to be undertaken lightly and I'd recommend that people think twice before embarking . . . all I'm prepared to say is that my subsequent nasal surgery has been entirely non-cosmetic.'

There are other problems about rhinoplasty. First of all, the shock of seeing a face so very different because of its different nose can sometimes be more than an individual has bargained for. One American woman was recently so disconcerted by her 'new look' that she said she needed 'psycho-cybernetics to adjust to my nose'.

The second problem, much more serious, often arises from unrealistic expectations about the results of surgery. It is not just that there is often a totally unreasonable fantasy about the beauty to come, but also that many women believe that surgery is not only going to alter their appearance, but that it will save their marriage, and improve and transform their whole personality. Worse still, as psychiatrists and surgeons freely admit, they have a constant queue of people who are suffering from serious psychological difficulties but who believe that cosmetic surgery will actually cure their neuroses and solve all life's problems. Inevitably, if they are operated on, such people are deeply disappointed and sink further into depression, even suicide. What is so often needed is not surgery but supportive counselling.

The trouble is that not all customers are able to explain exactly what it is they have in mind. The brave new nose of their imagination is beyond their powers of description, with the result that a surgeon may chisel away happily with an end-product in mind quite different from the dream nose of the client.

Standards of beauty, ideals of perfection, vary from individual to individual. And even more so from nation to nation. Australian aborigines, for example, have entirely different concepts of beauty from those in the West: they attempt to flatten the noses of their babies by pushing the child's head into the ground, or by constantly pressing the infant's nose with their hands. The last thing they want is the sharper aquiline nose of Europeans. Later on they may continue their strenuous efforts by piercing the septum – the central part of the nose – with a stick or bone to help spread the nose sideways and so bring about the squashed look so much desired.

In New Guinea external decoration is the important thing. Tusks and feathers are used to great effect to 'dress' the nose. Such ornaments are common in other countries too. To accommodate all manner of studs, chains and jewellery, holes are often pierced in the lower septum or in the nostrils. Valuable gold and diamond nose studs are especially popular on the Indian sub-continent. In the British Punk sub-culture, young men and women had less exotic but equally uncomfortable tastes, choosing to drape the nose with more utilitarian objects – preferably those with a hint of threat about them – like safety-pins, hooks or the occasional razor-blade.

Hooks in the nose were at one time also used in the Celebes, but for an entirely different reason. The nose was regarded as an important channel leading to the soul. Treatment of those who were sick often entailed plugging the nose to prevent the spirit departing prematurely. Alternatively, the nostrils of patients were lovingly pierced with fish hooks in an effort to capture the soul if it should be rash enough to attempt to escape.

EARMARKED

'Big ears', said Aristotle, are a sign that their owner has 'a tendency to irrelevant talk and chatter'. If this were so, then racial differences in ear sizes would define Asiatic, yellow/brown people – who have the largest ears – as talkative; and Africans – who have the smallest ears – as strong and silent. But character-analysis from ear shape and size is regarded with scepticism. Mr Spock, representing alien beings, seems appropriate enough with his pointed ears. In ancient legends the devil is always shown with sharply pointed ears. But serious assessments of character cannot be made from ears. Neither can any correlation be made between the shape and size of a face and the shape and size of its ears. A tiny, neat-featured person whose ears could reasonably be expected to be small might, like Chesterton's donkey, turn out to have 'ears like errant wings'.

Such a tempting flap of flesh could never have escaped unscathed from assaults in the name of beauty. The ear lobes especially present the most tempting and handiest places on which to hook ornamentation for the face. Western women have always been fond of ear pendants whose movements usually succeed in making the face look, by contrast, more serene. So if a still, immobile mask is wanted, then light-weight mobiles fluttering around the ears will certainly enhance this effect. For the energetic 'facialiser', however, a flurry of earrings against a busy face will contribute nothing at all to that particular, serene kind of beauty. For some people, vitality, liveliness and empathic facial movements may have more sympathetic appeal and appear more beautiful than the predictable monotony of a placid, static face.

There are some parts of the world where ears are used to keep personal treasure safe. In India, gold and jewelled earrings may easily represent a woman's fortune and may well be more secure in her ears than in her jewel box. In the South Pacific men and women are less concerned with storing up treasure in their ears, and much more interested in stretching their lobes to make them look attractive. The largest, most distended lobes are considered

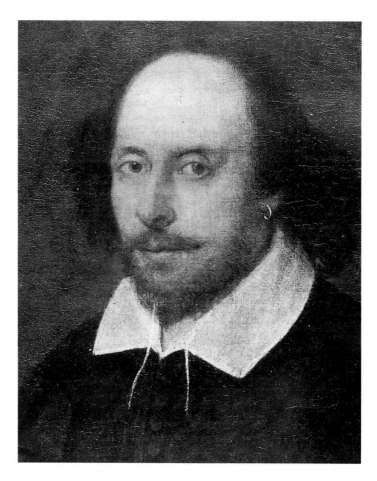

the best and all kinds of haberdashery are used to extend them: weighty knives and rings . . . even a half-smoked cigar. The anthropologist Sumner, early this century, saw one Melanesian woman with a little dog hanging to her ears by its feet. Such grotesque stretching can, however, prove a nuisance even to those who admire the dropped lobe. When forcing a way through hedge or bush, pendulous ears can get in the way, be torn, or even be ripped off.

Piercing of the ears has been popular for centuries. Shakespeare wore a single earring, and so did many of his contemporaries. Sailors long ago wore an earring as a talisman to ensure that they would be spared to come back to their loved one who was wearing the matching half of the pair. These days, piercing of a single ear has acquired some significance as a signal of homosexual preferences. Yet few seem reliably sure about which pierced ear denotes which affiliation. Is it the right ear or the left? The safest assumption is that if a male sports a single earring, he is not necessarily saying he is gay.

And Punks enjoyed multiple piercings: they would hang their protest jewellery from as many holes as their lobes could support. The fashion has since spread to more conventional, fashion-conscious people who have had their ears drilled all around the perimeter.

A B O V E : William Shakespeare sporting an earring

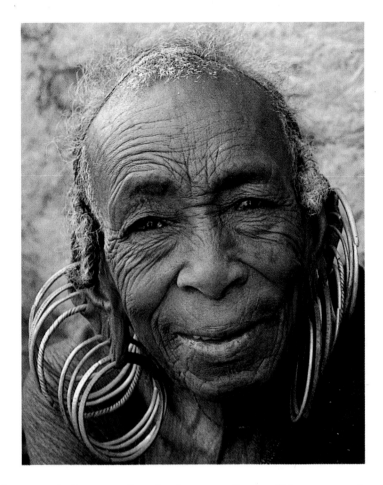

But even when carried out under the best sterile conditions, ear-piercing can cause infection. In 1988, Dr Peter Longstaff reported that he was seeing four or five patients a week – all with ears damaged as a result of piercing – in the Casualty Department of his London Hospital. Some ears are allergic to certain metals and it is common for an abscess to form. The ear lobes swell and both earring and a portion of the lobe often have to be removed *in toto*. Elderly women frequently have problems arising from piercing under-taken in their youth; the original holes enlarge and a corrective operation is needed. One woman, whose ears had been pierced for twenty-two years, found one day, while washing her hair, that one of her ear lobes had split. Her doctor referred her to a plastic surgeon who stitched it up again, for £280.

Now AIDS has raised a frightening spectre of infected needles. The popularity of ear-piercing is set for a decline in the 1990s with both men and women now much more cautious about the operation.

Among Oriental peoples the piercing of a young girl's ears was often a compulsory part of the initiation ritual which made her a woman in the eyes of her community. And sometimes the female ear has been regarded as a symbolic sexual orifice. It was for this

ABOVE: Nigerian woman with earrings galore

reason that, in ancient Egypt, slicing off the ears of an adulteress seemed appropriate punishment. In the same spirit mutilation of the ears has occasionally served, in some cultures, as an alternative for female circumcision. The Dogon women of Mali in North Africa, conscious of the sexual nature of the female ear, are particularly careful to wear earrings so as to protect their ears from evil intrusions. Zanzibar Omanis drill a hole through the back (rather than the lobe) of their ear so as not to let the djinn through. The djinn is the evil spirit which tries to enter the mind through the orifice of the ear but faced with this extra hole, enters through it instead and passes out again without causing trouble. In the West, texts on sexual techniques often stress the erotic effects of nibbling, stroking and kissing ears. At the Institute for Sex Research in Indiana, Kinsey and his team concluded that, occasionally, 'a female or male may reach orgasm as a result of stimulation of the ears'.

Really prominent, sticking-out ears have such an incongruous, unexpected quality that they often provoke unkind mirth, which can be psychologically damaging, especially for children. Some mothers are full of guilt and blame themselves for allowing their baby to sleep on a folded ear, which is certainly not the cause.

But the embarrassment of 'bat ears' is very real and the afflicted often seek help through plastic surgery. A crescent of skin from just behind the ear and a similar crescent from the ear flap can be removed and the two rear edges stitched together again. For men whose hair is short and for fastidious Punks whose Mohican hairstyles threw the ears into high relief, the effect on appearance can be dramatic. For children, the lifelong psychological benefits may be enormous.

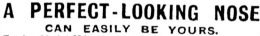
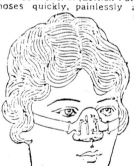
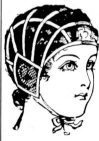

7. THE FACE:
CHANGING THE SHAPE

HOLDING AGE AT BAY

Tallulah Bankhead was not the first woman to make a mirror the scapegoat for her ageing face, when she commented that 'They're not making mirrors the way they used to!' Elizabeth I, appalled by her ruined reflection, banished mirrors from her Court altogether – whereupon the servants who made up her face each day took malicious advantage and painted her nose a cruel crimson.

The fact that youth's the stuff that won't endure is unhappily confirmed in the face. Contours change, colouring alters, chins multiply, jaws drop. Often, the face at seventy bears so little resemblance to the face at twenty that it would be easy to pass off a false identity.

But most people yearn to recover the smooth outlines of the face of youth. How we deal with this desire is up to us. We may decide to accept the inevitable and go nap on personality, or retreat into hiding, like Garbo, who withdrew from the public eye when her film days were over.

We may put up a fight against ageing by exploiting the arts of illusion– perhaps by framing the face more graciously with a softened hair-style, or by applying cunning make-up with a sleight of hand designed to deceive. Model girls have long known how to 'shape' their features with the help of a generous palette of cosmetic colours. Their finished faces are often the sculptured triumphs of tinted creams and powders and with never a surgeon's knife in sight.

Alternatively, we can attend Dr Ana Aslan's clinic to try her Gerovital H3 procaine-based youth treatment. 20,000 patients make the pilgrimage to Romania every year, yet more in the 73 countries where her drug is available – and despite medical argument – manage to have injections from their own doctor.

And then there is Dr Paul Niehans – patronised by the famous, and necessarily the very rich – who discovered 'Cell Therapy'. There are many who wish he had not discovered this disgusting treatment. His idea is this: the replacement cells for the millions we lose every second fall off in quality and quantity with age. So why not replace them with cells from unborn animals? Animals have the same biochemical structure as ourselves – sheep are particularly resistant to disease and, if foetus cells are used, they will be sterile and un-damaged. So the wombs are cut from these creatures, the embryos chopped while alive and the tissue cells immediately syringed into the patient. When Merle Oberon arrived for treatment she was approaching fifty – Niehan said she would soon feel twenty. After a week she reported favourable results – more energy, glowing skin, body tight and strong. Much the same reaction, in fact, that those who have taken Royal Jelly report. Manufactured by worker bees from a gland in their head to feed the developing queen bee, Royal Jelly is presently under scrutiny by Professor Robinson of King's College, at the University of London. 96% of Royal Jelly's constituents are known and there is nothing remarkable about them. But there remains an elusive, tantalizing 4% which defies analysis. So is it just a folk medicine for people who like to believe in what Dr Tom Sanders has recently called 'fairies at the bottom of the bottle'? Or is it really Cliff Richard's secret of youthfulness? Or even that of the Princess of Wales, the Duchess of York, Barbara Cartland and Millwall football team all of whom are said to be consumers of Royal Jelly? It is certainly the 'bees-knees' in China, Japan, Greece and all over the Eastern bloc where – according to Mrs Irene Stein, founder of 'Regina' Jelly – they take it seriously. Honey can certainly do no harm – unless it happens to be the so-called 'Mad Honey' from Turkey which the *Journal of the American Medical Association* says causes blood pressure to fall and the heart to slow down. Nectar from *Rhododendron ponticum* is the culprit.

Another much talked-about treatment was an amorphous powder prepared from the posterior lobes of the mammalian pituitary gland. A muscular energiser, it activated the pressor muscles and was found useful in increasing the pushing movement during labour. It also increased blood pressure and acted as an anti-diuretic. Developed by Swiss clinics as a general rejuvenator and known as 'Monkey Gland', it was all the rage in the 1920s.

Of all the options, cosmetic surgery is the one which is increasing the fastest, especially in the United States. There, 600,000 men and women are holding age at bay on a knife-edge. One New Yorker who began with eyelid surgery now goes regularly every year to her surgeon for a retread (her doctor prefers to call it a 'sequel'). She captures the modern mood exactly: 'Why let the bit of extra skin show on your face when you wouldn't permit it anywhere else?' she asks. Her philosophy is simple and straightforward; if anything is slipping, sagging or falling about, then have it put right.

For her, the money is available and so is the manpower to do the job. In the United States surgeons are plentiful: in one state alone, for a population of three million there are fifty-two qualified plastic surgeons. In Britain, by contrast, for a population of 55 million there are only 150 who are fully qualified. And this may account in some part for the difference in attitudes, although Dr Gerald Imber in New York still believes that Britons are much too inhibited and 'draw an altogether stupid line about how far they are prepared to go to look good'.

There are exceptions however. For Maria Kay, a BBC sound engineer in her mid-thirties and someone not in the public eye, cosmetic plastic surgery is her hobby. As she mentioned in an interview in the magazine *She* (in July 1988), 'when you alter one thing it has a knock-on effect'. She had had two nose operations and may have a tiny bit more off still. She has had also collagen implants in her forehead, and she intends to have more silicone cheek-bones implanted: 'The right one is slightly squiffy – but I bashed my

OPPOSITE: How has Joan Collins (who disapproves of cosmetic surgery) kept age at bay so successfully?

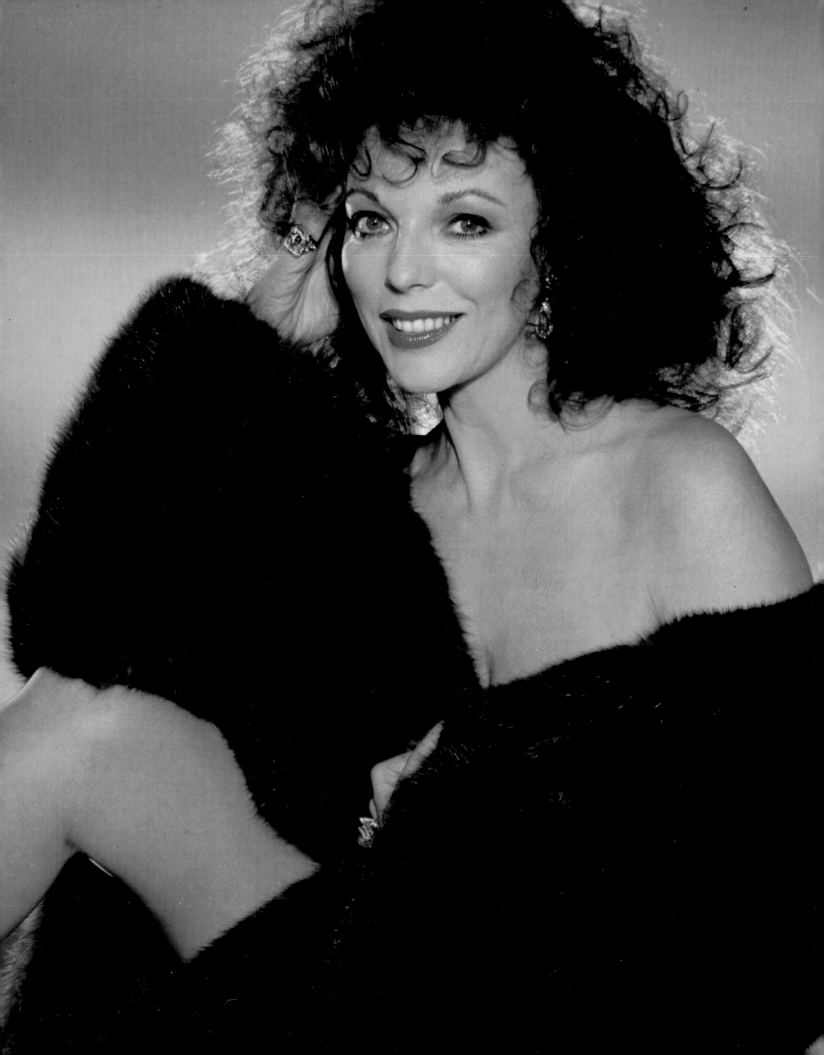

knee against it when I was pottering around my plants so I probably caused it. It's quite painful afterwards because your jaw feels dislocated – it's very stiff – and you have to go on a liquid diet for five days. Food particles can cause infection if they catch in the stitches but you can't chew anyway. You can't smile. Your face aches. . . .'

She has had dermabrasion and will carry on having it.

Later on she will have a 'voluptuous' new lip-line tattooed, plus tattooed eyebrows (her own never grew again properly after over-plucking). In a few months' time, she will have chemical peeling to get rid of wrinkles. Chemical peeling will mean sleeping sitting up for a month to help the bruising. 'It's so poisonous . . . you can't risk it getting into the bloodstream.'

After all this she will have buttock and thigh tucks.

'It's all purely for myself. I am an idealist and would like to look what I consider to be aesthetically perfect.'

Americans have no hesitation in putting right any of Nature's tactless reminders of advancing years. If a husband leaves you, don't pine, have a face-lift, is the advice. It seems to work: one septuagenarian who underwent surgery describes herself as full of new purpose and joie-de-vivre. Now that she is over the shock, she says she is quite glad to be rid of her 83 year-old absconder.

With enviable candour American women will usually readily disclose which of their parts have been reconditioned, or perhaps even replaced. As to the identity of their surgeons, there is little point in trying to keep this secret. In fact, many believe that the hall-mark of individual surgeons can be readily detected. As David Niven put it: 'You can tell a woman's plastic surgeon by the cut of her.'

Those more diffident about revealing it can always fly down to Rio where Dr Ivo Pitanguy – described in an article in *You* as 'the world's best surgeon' – offers sanctuary as well as surgery. With 40,000 operations to his credit he leaves no trade-mark on his work, save the stamp of perfection. And he is discreetly non-committal when it comes to naming his famous patients. But he does reveal that the most common request he has is for facial surgery to defeat ageing.

In the States, having a face-lift is becoming commonplace. But 'face-lift' is, of course, only an umbrella term; as surgeons point out, the individual problems of the face vary from person to person. So while removing a double chin may be a major part of one individual's face-lift, for another, lifting the brow may be the most important objective.

Some take to their lifts more happily than others. Men and women with high cheek-bones have an advantage because their bony framework helps to hold up the manipulated skin. Those less fortunately structured can overcome this by having implants – artificial cheekbones made of silicone – a good investment since these false cheek-bones may double the life of their lift.

And when does a 'lift' need to become a 'hoist'? Usually when brow furrows and vertical lines between the eyes begin to resist the blandishments of the scalpel. A conventional face-lift will pull the skin upwards and so remove brow wrinkles quite satisfactorily, but these forehead 'expression lines' tend to be annoyingly persistent and may well be back again within a year – especially for those people who use their faces vigorously to communicate. So some surgeons penetrate deeper into the flesh and cut into the glabella muscle. This way the lines will disappear more permanently though you, the patient, will no longer be able to frown at all.

There are, though, one or two other dangers worth mentioning, like the possibility of prolonged numbness from nerve damage which may last sometimes for a year or more, and also the danger of over-correction which can result in a 'terribly surprised expression'.

New methods are constantly being explored: the scope for structural change seems limitless. Faces can now be reshaped not only by lifting the skin and introducing collagen, but by implanting silicone, and even bone and cartilage too. This latter technique is a spin-off from the world of restorative and accident surgery. But it is being used more and more to fulfil aesthetic ambitions, both reasonable and unreasonable.

Another method, showing great promise, though not yet fully tested, is a kind of 'Peter and Paul' technique known as autologous fat grafting, in which fat which may be readily spared from hips or from buttocks, or even thighs, is introduced into the face in areas which need filling out.

Even the conventional face-lift, where the skin is slit, and lifted up in front of the ears, has been overtaken in the USA. There is now a 'double-layered face-lift'. Like the creators of restorative creams, surgeons have turned their attention to that criss-crossed dermis layer which lies below the epidermal surface of the skin. Putting a tuck in the surface skin is all very well, they point out, but if the tissue below is in disorder, then the improvement may last only a few months.

In the double-layered face-lift – or SMAS-lift (the 'suprafacial musculo-aponeurotic system') – the surgeon works on the subcutaneous muscle and fat below the surface skin, as well as the surface skin itself. And whilst temporary numbness and swelling and possible nerve injury are taken for granted in both types of operation, it is SMAS which carries an even greater danger of nerve injury – even permanent paralysis of the facial muscles.

THE FACE OF DISCONTENT

Clearly, any woman or man contemplating facial surgery should spend time carefully investigating the credentials of a prospective surgeon. Success is much more likely in the hands of a qualified surgeon who is a member of a reputable professional body such as the British Association of Plastic Surgeons or the British Association of Aesthetic Surgeons.

Operators in some of the widely advertised clinics may not be specially qualified at all. The British Medical Association has a bulging dossier of complaints from patients who have suffered post-operative complications such as infection, or who have been left scarred, or worse still, disabled.

Recently, in Britain, a middle-aged woman needed four hours of extra surgery for her face-lift and had to have a hole cut in her throat to help her breathe. Her cosmetic improvements turned out to be a life-and-death struggle – for which she was charged £2,400.

In Britain, anyone at all can perform cosmetic surgery provided it is on human beings, not animals, but as one consultant plastic surgeon said recently: 'The cosmetic surgery world is in desperate need of policing.' Dr Ian Todd, President of the Royal College of Surgeons, has explained the official attitude: 'The only people we recognise as capable of carrying out cosmetic surgery operations are plastic surgeons who have gained our Fellowship and then a further certificate of accreditation from us. The others are simply cowboys.'

Unfortunately, there are a lot of cowboys about – and they are prospering. High pressure advertising and selling methods are tempting people into what turn out to be little more than back-street clinics hired for the week-end, where rushed operations are performed, usually without adequate prior investigation or counselling – and without any kind of after-care. The companies aiding and abetting these surgeons are all too ready to give their dubious advice on how to raise the money which, in one recently reported case was: 'Tell your bank manager you need a personal loan to buy a new car.'

Quick profits in this high-growth area seem too tempting to resist. A disgraced plastic surgeon in Glasgow in 1987 recommended a private hospital in which he had shares to the parents of a seven-year-old boy for the removal of a blemish on his lip. Complications developed, the surgeon did not call in help soon enough and the little boy died. In 1985, a nurse whose life was being made a misery by cruel taunts about her looks died after cosmetic surgery to remove her double chin. There were problems with a drainage tube in her chin and she suffered a heart attack.

Vogue, which in 1987 surveyed the whole field of cosmetic surgery, concluded: 'All cosmetic operations carry the risk of infection and bad scarring.'

Indeed, all surgery has its risks which for life-threatening conditions are readily accepted. The tragic mutilations from warfare, road accidents, burns, birthmarks or the unearned saddle-nose of congenital syphilis – all of which now yield to surgical treatment – are worth taking risks to remove. Whether to take chances for the vanity of appearing to be younger than one's true age is something for each individual to decide. The assumption that a younger face will create a younger spirit or a renewed zest for living may be misguided. As Dr Pitanguy has pointed out, to look young you have to feel young inside, and this does not always come by removing the wrinkles of age: 'If someone believes we can restore youth, they have a problem.'

An even greater and much more dangerous problem arises when the applicant for surgery has an undefined discontent and cannot express what seems to be the trouble. Or when there is a fixation that a certain feature, for some mysterious reason, is 'wrong'. Time and a psychologist are needed to unravel these problems, and well before any surgeon reaches for his scalpel. Quite frequently, even the most elegant and well-endowed have irrational pangs of uncertainty about their appearance and are harshly critical of their own faces. Often enough this springs from deeper worries and doubts about the person inside and masks a desperation which will not be relieved by surgery. Conscientious surgeons who sense that a prospective patient's unhappiness about outward appearance is really a thinly veiled dissatisfaction with the self beneath will usually suspend operations until motivations and attitudes have been investigated further.

Again, we may need to square with ourselves a certain feeling of loss of strength of character. We have not been able to stand up to looking older. We have gone into hiding behind a mask of pretend youth. We have also stepped outside the expectations of our age group. Nowadays many over-sixties are running companies; some are Prime Ministers. But there is a certain borderline of decorum which, if crossed, tends to bring down the resentment of those younger ones who feel that one has gone too far, overstepped the mark, forgotten just how old one really is. And this resentment – unjust though it may be – needs to be lived down and coped with.

Men can be more sensitive than women in this difficult area of 'acting one's age'. Uncertainties and anxieties about vigour and virility are easily raised.

It is not just age that breeds in us discontent with our faces. People in the prime of life are susceptible too. In the United States where requests for facial surgery have doubled since 1982 there are now many more patients between thirty-five and fifty-four.

That the mid-thirties is a good time to start is the opinion of Bernard Kaye, Clinical Professor of Plastic Surgery at the University of Florida. Career-driven men and women in the public eye and high-flyers of the business world often feel they have a need to look alert and fit and attractive. In Britain – in these competitive days – little store is placed on the sagacity and experience of the elderly. In America, 'AARP' (The American Association of Retired Persons) with 29 million members, has broken free of this downbeat image of age. A president well into his seventies has been proof enough that there can be meaningful life-after-sixty. And this may well contribute to the feeling in the United States that it is worth while rehabilitating the ageing face, whatever the age.

Film stars and stage performers certainly feel they owe it to their audiences to be attractive. When Tom Jones was asked if he would ever have more surgery he said yes, he would if it became necessary to sustain his image as a star. It was part of the job.

Oscar-winning actress Cher – who has spent £24,000 on plastic surgery – makes no secret of her attitude: 'When there's a bit of me I don't like, I change it.' She has had her cheek-bones shaped up, her nose slimmed down and shortened, her acne scars removed and her chin modified by silicone implant.

Marilyn Monroe felt that her jaw was wrong and her nose needed to be re-shaped. Even after she had had these problems dealt with by surgery she still had the idea that the distance between her nose and upper lip was really too short. To compensate for this she took care to speak with her upper lip pouting downwards, a habit which – as it happened – became one of the hall-marks of her appealing 'sex-kitten' style.

What Marilyn was seeking for herself was a face which would satisfy impossible notions of a perfect beauty and sexual attractiveness drummed up by producers, directors and publicity departments. Joan Crawford too underwent painful and totally unnecessary dentistry simply to alter the shape of her jaw in pursuit of studio ideals. And the whim of fashion can sometimes bring about a short-lived demand for some particular feature or characteristic. Western beauties in magazines and on the screen ape the exotica of other – even ancient – civilisations and create novelty and temporary styles which others strenuously attempt to follow. In the 1960s, in homage to Elizabeth Taylor, a thousand suburban Cleopatras lined their eyes, straightened their hair and then dyed it Egyptian black.

Occasionally this process happens in reverse and beauties of other lands are influenced by Western standards, making almond eyes round, black skins white and curly hair straight.

In the feverish urge to comply with a currently fashionable ideal, even the skull has not escaped manipulations of various kinds. In Nazi Germany, worried parents used to massage their babies' heads in an effort to remove any last traces of decadent Mediterra-nean roundness, and to transform them into the long, much-favoured Aryan shape so characteristic of the 'Master Race'. In Holland, at one time, the tight-fitting cap worn by females all their lives – and by boys up to the age of seven or eight – was regarded as having the advantage of improving the shape of the skull.

In France too, there was once the custom of restricting upward growth of the heads of newborn children with a tight bandeau of linen which produced the highly desirable effect of flattening the skull. The children cried for hours, the bandage was seldom removed, harboured lice and frequently gave rise to skin infections and ulcers.

But this skull deformation is by no means a European monopoly; there are many tribes who have made a practice of lengthening, shortening, widening or narrowing the heads of their children in order to achieve some purely local ideal of excellence. American Indians for many centuries tied boards to their babies' heads to produce an 'ideal' shape. Mangbettu women of Central Africa who admired a cone-shaped head used to press their babies' heads between pieces of giraffe hide tied tightly around the skull.

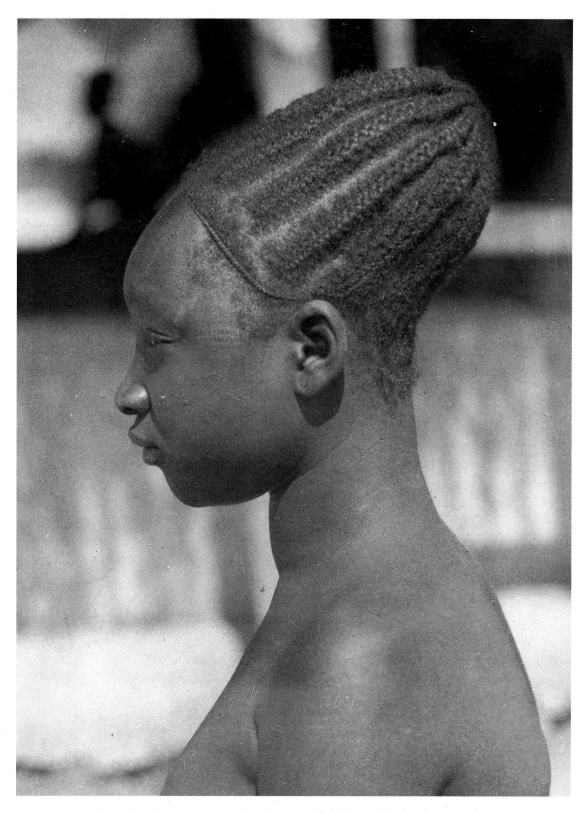

This Mangbettu woman's head was artificially moulded to its cone shape

Hippocrates and Pliny wrote about the popularity of head deformation which usually started at birth, in high-born families of ancient Greece and Rome. The ancient Egyptians also had very clear ideas about the 'perfect' head shape, hence the famous, elongated head of Nefertiti. Such is the flexibility of the human organism that there appears to have been little damage to brain function. Indeed, the Mangbettu believed that the desirable cone-shape encouraged greater intelligence.

In the seventeenth and eighteenth centuries, women in Britain had their own unique, non-surgical method of shoring up their faces. They used 'plumpers', small round balls made of cork or leather. These uncomfortable objects – often as much as two and a half inches in diameter – were slipped into the mouth to push outwards the collapsed flesh of the cheeks. Salesmen offered them with the cheery cry: 'Take heart the hang-toothed and drop-cheeked, for our Plumpers can fill up the cavities of your cheeks' – a tempting message indeed in those days of neglected teeth, early decay and the very common problem of 'resorption', the shrinking of the jaws which happens in old age or after teeth have fallen out. Many women who wore these devices found themselves in difficulties with their speech. Some of them mastered the art of talking through their plumpers by making delicate sucking movements. The final effect produced a lisping style of speech which, though initially a disadvantage, eventually became quite fashionable and was much admired in genteel ladies.

But alas, some ladies never quite conquered the technique of wearing their plumpers; many wore them but failed to manage even a lisp. They were obliged to keep silent, preferring to look well rather than run the risk of sounding less than well. As Mrs Cowley in *The Beaux' Stratagem* explained: 'Mrs Button wears cork plumpers in each cheek and never hazards more than six words for fear of showing them.'

Whether to wear plumpers, to have a face-lift, an implant, a tuck here or a tuck there, or to leave well alone is every human being's right of choice. Who can dictate how we should or should not decorate or even refashion our faces? The bliss of removing a flaw that has given a lifetime of sleepless nights and reduced self-confidence to zero may be felt to be worth any amount of risk, discomfort and expense.

Women, at any rate, have never questioned that at least some of their flaws can be dealt with. In the present century, the conviction that an offending feature can be cajoled, bullied and generally whipped into shape is being reaffirmed daily. So much more is possible, and no longer just for the wealthy. The 'knifestyles of the rich and famous', as *You* magazine coined the phrase, has become a boom industry with more and more available for men and women of quite modest means. Scalpels are at the ready for the creation of designer faces. If the present rate of progress continues, if surgery and vanity succeed in keeping pace with each other, how long will it be before we contemplate spare parts surgery for the face? Nowadays, nothing seems too remote, too drastic or too dangerous. When personal beauty is at stake there are no holds barred.

8. CROWNS OF GLORY: THE HAIR

Hair is the most important complement to the face. Its shape, colour and texture form the face's frame and considerably alter how we perceive the face's features and also its size. Hair fashions have always changed as constantly as the seasons. Springing out from our heads, and growing an inch a month until it reaches ten inches then slowing down by half, hair is also capable of being coloured, cut and contoured to taste, giving us scope to make significant non-verbal declarations of all kinds. By fashioning it appropriately, we can signal a generation gap, tell the world what group we belong to or wish to belong to, show defiance or submission, indicate mood, invite or repel. The langorous act of unpinning long hair and allowing it to cascade to the waist, or even to the shoulder, has never quite gone out of fashion as an act of sexual invitation, or submission.

A BURNING BEAUTY: CHANGING THE SHADE

Toyah Willcox had her hair mistaken for a hat by MGM's film director George Cukor when she was at the height of her psychedelic glory in 1981. She had sprayed, dyed and fanned it out into shapes and colours more extravagant than the headdress of a Busby Berkeley girl. Before her, the Punks had already set the standard for sculpted, rainbow-coloured hair. And twenty years before them, Wee Willie Harris had trail-blazed by dyeing his hair a candy-floss pink which dripped down his collar in the rain. Tiger Morse had changed the colour of her hair eighteen times in eighteen months and Zandra Rhodes had streaked her hair cerise, orange, blue and green. But dyeing and bleaching hair was not exclusive to women. Andy Warhol had set the trend in the early Sixties, closely followed by David Hockney and then David Bowie who gave it the final seal of approval. For men, women, and the undecided, coloured hair – the more unnatural the better – was the new excitement.

It was in the Seventies with the followers of the new Punk movement that exotic hairstyles reached their peak. Anti-establishment, anti-Royal, anti-nature and pro-artifice, the Punks established their identity most strenuously through their hair. To shock was essential, and no combination of cut and colour was considered too extraordinary. The subdued greys of overcast streets were suddenly ablaze with heads as vibrant as sarees in a paddy field. Topiaried hairstyles, in every hue, walked the parks and challenged the flowers. No need for Punks to be vocal: their hair, their most versatile accomplice, did their talking for them.

But hair has its breaking point. Lillie Langtry, a mistress of Edward, Prince of Wales, had her hair dyed by the Austrian Court hairdresser and, to her horror, finished up with

EDWARDS' "HARLENE" FOR THE HAIR

The Great Hair Producer and Restorer.

The Finest Dressing. Specially Prepared and Delicately Perfumed. A Luxury and a Necessity to every Modern Toilet.

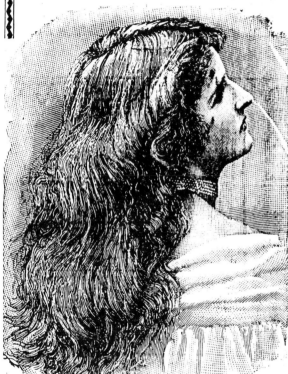

Under Royal Patronage and Supplied direct to

H.M. THE QUEEN OF GREECE.
H.I.H. THE GRAND DUCHESS GEORGE OF RUSSIA.
H.R.H. PRINCESS HOHENLOHE.
H.R.H. THE DUKE OF SPARTA.
H.H. PRINCESS WINDISCHGRAETZ.
H.R.H. THE DUCHESS OF SPARTA.
H.I.H. THE GRAND DUCHESS OF MECKLENBURG-SCHWERIN.
H.I.H. PRINCE GEORGE OF GREECE.
H.H. PRINCESS DI SIPINO.
PRINCESS ANNA HOHENLOHE, etc.

Restores, Strengthens, Beautifies, and Promotes the Growth of the Hair.

PREVENTS ITS FALLING OFF AND TURNING GREY.

The World-renowned Cure for Baldness.

Miss JULIA NEILSON

writes: "I am at present trying your 'HARLENE' for my hair and I find it one of the best hair tonics and restorers I have ever used, and I have tried many."

Mrs. LANGTRY writes:

"Previous to using 'HARLENE' my Hair had become brittle, and was falling off. I have used your preparation daily for eighteen months, and my hair is quite restored. I cannot recommend 'HARLENE' too highly."

A FREE TRIAL BOTTLE	Will be sent to any part of the world to any person filling up this form and enclosing 3d. for postage (Foreign stamps accepted). If presented personally at our offices, no charge will be made.
	Name..
	Address...

HOME NOTES (Nov. 16, 1905)

1/-, 2/3, and 4/6 per Bottle, from Chemists and Stores all over the world, or sent direct on receipt of Postal Orders.

EDWARDS' "HARLENE" CO., 95 & 96 High Holborn, London, W.C.

DEPILATORIES.

As recipes for these are frequently sought, we give the following: (1) One hundred grains of sulphide of soda; eighty grains of slaked lime; twenty grains of starch; four fluid drachms of lime water. (2) Eighty grains of barium sulphide; four hundred grains of powdered chalk.

The first recipe is for a paste, to be used without further addition of water. The second recipe is for a powder. To use this a small quantity must be made into paste with water immediately before it is to be applied.

(3) Two drachms of sulphide of strontium; three drachms of oxide of zinc; three drachms of powdered starch. To be made into a paste as stated above.

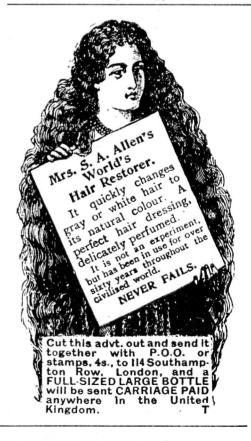

blonde hair alternating with violent stripes of heliotrope, obliging her, for some time, to wear a wig.

Henri III of France became prematurely bald as a result of trying to dye his hair, and for years wore a wig or a turban.

For hundreds of years women have attempted to bleach their hair, often disastrously.

But tradition has it that to be blonde is to be beautiful. Accounts of perfect women always rhapsodised on spun gold hair: Shakespeare's 'golden net to entrap the hearts of men faster than gnats in cobwebs'. In traditional folk stories, fairy queens have almost always been blonde and witches dark. And this ideal of blonde perfection persists throughout medieval literature. In fact there are very few black-haired maidens in literature from Homer to Shakespeare, as one classical scholar has observed. American sociologists, Utter and Needham, agree. In their recent study of working-girl novels of the nineteenth century, eighty out of a hundred heroines were blonde, only ten were brunette and ten had red hair.

Modern film stars have continued the tradition. Marilyn Monroe was a natural brunette, but with remarkable commercial prescience studio chiefs bleached her hair to palest platinum.

Madonna, blue-eyed and Harlow-blonde and considered by many to be Marilyn's successor, suddenly appeared with surprisingly dark hair in David Mamet's 1988 play, *Speed-the-Plow*. In this reincarnation as a brunette, the critics' consensus was that 'she looks sexier than ever'. However, for this self-styled 'Material Girl', it may have been more of a practical solution. Already Madonna had been forced into a shorter hairstyle: the American hair salon Bumble and Bumble said she was suffering from serious 'hair fall out' due to so much bleaching.

Women – and men – have all too often paid a high price for their bleachings and dyeings. Roman women tried to imitate the hair dyes and bleaches used by the Gauls. But the hair of the ancient Romans had neither the quality nor coarse strength of Germanic tresses and instead of turning pale, it just dropped out altogether. Still covetous of the golden look, enraged and balding Roman ladies then demanded that the hair of the Gauls be cut off and made into wigs for themselves. The idea had about it a certain piquancy and was said to have met with Caesar's enthusiastic approval: chopping off the hair of a nation they had conquered and parading it publicly on victorious Roman heads was a humiliation entirely to his taste.

There have been occasions, however, when some ladies have favoured black hair. When their natural hair had become grey, ancient Egyptians and Romans, for example, settled for dark hair. The Egyptians used a mixture which included the blood of a black cow, tortoise-shell and the neck of the gabgu-bird, cooked in oil; another favourite recipe required the womb of a cat. And Pliny described one old Roman recipe which specified a pint of leeches and two quarts of pure vinegar pounded and fermented for sixty days. But he added the grave warning that when this mixture was finally rubbed into the scalp, it was important to hold oil in the mouth otherwise teeth, too, would go black.

Some alert ladies in the seventeenth century noticed that when hair was wet it reacted with lead and became black. So lead combs were pressed into service for darkening the hair. The inevitable side-effect, however, was not realised at the time: lead was poisonous – even lethal. When absorbed into the scalp in sufficient amounts, it can soon cause kidney disease.

Two centuries later, renewed experimentation led to another theory: since dark hair was probably caused by an excess of iron in the system, then acids to neutralise the iron might well be successful in lightening the hair. What was recommended was an ounce of pure oxalic acid – which happens to be a strong poison – mixed with a pint of boiling water, allowed to cool a little and then sponged on to the head. This should be followed by a thorough drying out in sunlight. The procedure could be repeated: 'until it begins to affect the skin when it must be discontinued, otherwise the hair will fall out'.

Fewer problems today for Ronald Reagan perhaps: general gossip has it that he uses the ready-made Grecian 2000 which boasts that it will not 'shock' the hair with harsh chemicals (it contains no peroxide) but will gently, gradually 'coax' the hair back to its natural colour. Care is still needed. Grecian 2000's formula includes lead acetate. Hands should be carefully washed after using it, and it should not be used on an irritated or broken scalp.

The desire to produce colours other than black for the hair was always more difficult to satisfy. Hair powders were tried, though unpleasantly heavy greasing with its risk of putrefaction was required if the powder was to stick to the hair. Vegetable dyes were sometimes used: in medieval times, for instance, crushed saffron was employed to yellow the hair.

In Venice in the nineteenth century ladies took to bleaching their hair by first soaking it in caustic solutions, then spreading their hair in the sun until it obediently turned yellow, or – as all too frequently happened – dropped out. An alternative suggestion recommended: 'A paste of bisulphate of magnesia and lime is very effectual in bleaching the hair', but added the somewhat jaunty warning, 'and also for burning it away entirely, together with the skin and brains, if there are any, beneath it'.

In Britain, women used this formula and then attempted to colour their hair yellow with solutions of cadmium, arsenic or gold. The arsenic was usually in the form of orpiment or realgar, both deadly in their cumulative effect. Yet this particular brace of poisons was destined to form the base for the majority of golden hair dyes for a great number of years to come. Many cases of poisoning were reported in the newspapers of the nineteenth century.

OPPOSITE : Punks established their identity most strenuously through their hair

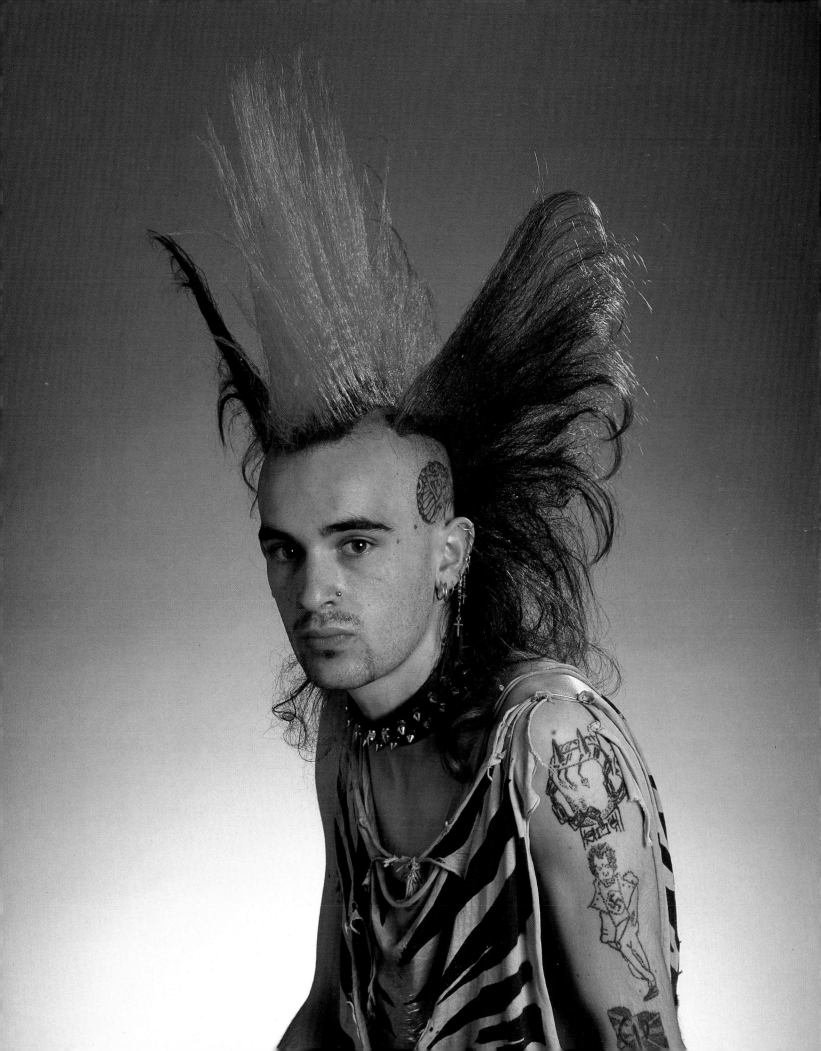

The hair designer Raymond in more recent times found that he could turn hair ash blonde by bleaching it and then colouring it with strong coffee or tea, adding a discreet drop or two of oil of cloves – presumably to mask the smell. It was only in 1946 that Clairol developed more scientifically-based colourings and Raymond abandoned his highly original tinting methods.

But Raymond's solutions did have the advantage of being unquestionably safe and wholesome. Not that the safety aspect of hair care has ever been a matter of much concern to the thousands of women, and the growing number of men too, who regularly dye their hair. Few of us think about the long-term effects of hair dyes when we drop our willing heads into the salon bowl. As the hairdresser Annie Russell pointed out, 'Most women don't realise how destructive even shampoo can be'.

In the United States, after customers complained of eye irritation, a group of shampoos was discovered to be responsible for clouding of the cornea. Resorcinol, a common constituent of anti-dandruff shampoos and a powerful antiseptic, was found to be damaging the delicate tissues of the eyes.

Even bad breath can result from the use of shampoos containing Selenium sulphide; 'tremor, perspiration and pain in the lower abdomen' have also been reported.

Hair colourants – of which there are three major kinds – need even greater care in use than do shampoos. The simplest are temporary rinses which coat the shaft of the hair without penetrating it. They wash out readily, but this is not such good news if you are caught out in the rain.

Semi-permanent hair colourants, best used to darken the hair, are more long-lasting. They slightly penetrate the hair shafts as well as coating them and usually last about six weeks. But there can be allergic reactions which tend to affect the scalp. There may be unpleasant swelling, itching and oozing of the skin. Medication too can cause reactions: one hairdresser found black patches emerging on a client's scalp during colouring. It turned out that the lady's 'tablets' were to blame – a perverse and unpleasant synergic reaction.

Permanent hair colouring – probably best undertaken at a salon because of the importance of timing and other technical problems – often involves the removal of existing colour – e.g. the brunette who is changing to blonde. The dye is mixed with the bleach – hydrogen peroxide – but if carelessly left on for too long the hair can be made so brittle that it will break off and fall away.

'But the real nightmare', said one hairdresser, 'is when a client has coloured her hair at home and then comes straightaway to us for a perm'. Dr Vernon Coleman confirms this: 'If you subject your hair to a permanent wave and a permanent colourant at the same time then you really ought to have a wig ready in the wardrobe.'

In 1975, a warning about toxic absorption came from the Biochemistry department of the University of California: 'surprisingly little has been published about the absorption of the various components of hair dyes through the skin of the human scalp'. And in 1977 *The British Medical Journal* added the further warning that many dyes were strongly mutagenic. In the States, where 20 million women dye their hair regularly, there has been concern about one particular toxic ingredient, diaminotoluene, known to be cancer-producing when fed to rats, which has been banned from hair dyes since 1971. *The Lancet*, in a survey of 120,557 nurses in the States, demonstrated a statistically significant association between the use of permanent hair dye and the development of cancer of the cervix.

In their valuable 1985 'survey of surveys' of undesirable side-effects of cosmetic products, Nater and de Groot found that hair colourants and bleaches were among the 'top six' troublemakers in no less than three separate enquiries. There were nearly 10,000 instances recorded of unpleasant reactions. Hair straighteners too, they investigated, and classified as 'high risk' products. The Royal Cancer Hospital, London, has warned that 'the experimental evidence that many hair dye constituents are mutagenic and that some are carcinogenic is irrefutable'. In 1978, however, a Mr Van Abbé discounted such fears saying that repeated dyeing was unlikely to cause any greater chromosomal damage than, for example, routine dental X-rays. But his argument seemed less impressive when it was discovered that he was associated with a cosmetic manufacturer.

Controversy about the extent of possible adverse effects of hair dyes continues. But women, understandably, will not readily be dissuaded from touching up their hair. Greying hair is a universal horror, especially those first few aggressive tufts which spring from the scalp indecently proclaiming the advancing years.

For HM Customs and Immigration the task of keeping up with changing shades has evidently proved too much. In 1969 they told us that it was no longer necessary to declare the colour of our hair on British passports. The final proof perhaps, that the colour of hair is too difficult to keep up with and the desire for change too powerful an instinct to cope with.

FRIZZING AND GLUEING: CHANGING THE SHAPE

A young woman asked to see her hairdresser privately, and arrived wearing a turban and in a state of distress. The hair on her head was an all-over fuzz of no more than half an inch long. The rest was in a plastic bag. She had attempted to bleach it with a paste made up of Domestos and Vim (household bleach and scouring powder). This, after a perm less than two days old. 'And I only left it on for a few minutes,' she said.

Even bleaches specifically designed for the task can weaken the shafts of the hair, make it more porous and if used excessively make it brittle enough to break. To follow a bleach immediately with a perm or vice-versa is a formula for disaster.

All hairdressers have their horror stories of women who have attempted to tint their hair themselves straight after a perm and who have found that there is more of it left on the pillow than on their head. An even greater nightmare is the client who has been treated at the salon but whose hair has reacted badly to perming or straightening. Vidal Sassoon, in his very early apprenticeship, forgot to turn off the power and left a client under a 'perm machine' during an air raid. When the 'all clear' sounded, her hairdo was nicely crisped. Fortunately – during those give-and-take wartime days – all was forgiven.

Curling, waving, shaping the hair to create a flattering frame for the face is something most women will attempt at some time in their lives. How we arrange our hair can make such a profound difference to the face. A high, wide hairstyle, for example, can render a woman's face more petite and therefore more feminine.

If we decide to permanently wave our hair we must, however, first of all structurally damage it. Lotions – usually the thioglycolates – are applied to the hair to disrupt the chemical bonding; then new shapes are created by winding the now-flexible hair around curlers. After a precise time the hair is rinsed, and then neutralised either by letting it oxidise naturally or by using a solution which contains an oxidising agent, for example, hydrogen peroxide. The timing is crucial. Brittle, 'frizzed' hair is the penalty for leaving waving lotions on too long or failing to neutralise properly.

Many women these days turn to perms not so much for tight curls but to give more body to their hair. In 1988 L'Oréal introduced their 'Jetting Perm' – designed to be without curl but with 'body and lift' and said to last about six weeks.

Not everyone wants curls. Quite the reverse. There was a time when black performers of stage and television used to grease their naturally curly hair and then attempt to straighten it with the help of products such as the 'Yvette Home Hair Straightening Kit'.

Hot combs were also used. As one young man from Africa explained recently, it was a 'round the fireside' job. 'We used to do my sister's hair at home. We put the comb in the fire or the gas and made it very hot. Then we took a strand or two of her hair and ran the hot comb along it.'

More sophisticated efforts do not always meet with success. The combined use of hot combs and chemical solutions like sodium hydroxide or lye are capable of burning hair away if used incorrectly. When this happened to Shirley Bassey she sued the company she held responsible.

In the late 1960s when black finally became beautiful, there was a sudden cross-cultural swing, and Western fashion embraced the traditional hairstyles of Africa and the Caribbean. Women and men demanded bushy 'Afro' styles. Rastafarian dread-locks dangled atop Marks and Spencer tee-shirts. Matted hair and all the Rasta accoutrements of rings, bracelets and spectacular sun-glasses were taken up by pop stars. Superstars Bob Marley and Eddy Grant exemplified the look. Europeans were dazzled by it but achieved

OPPOSITE : Cornrowing and beadwork from (*top*) Zimbabwe, (*bottom left*) Gabon, and (*bottom right*) Senegal

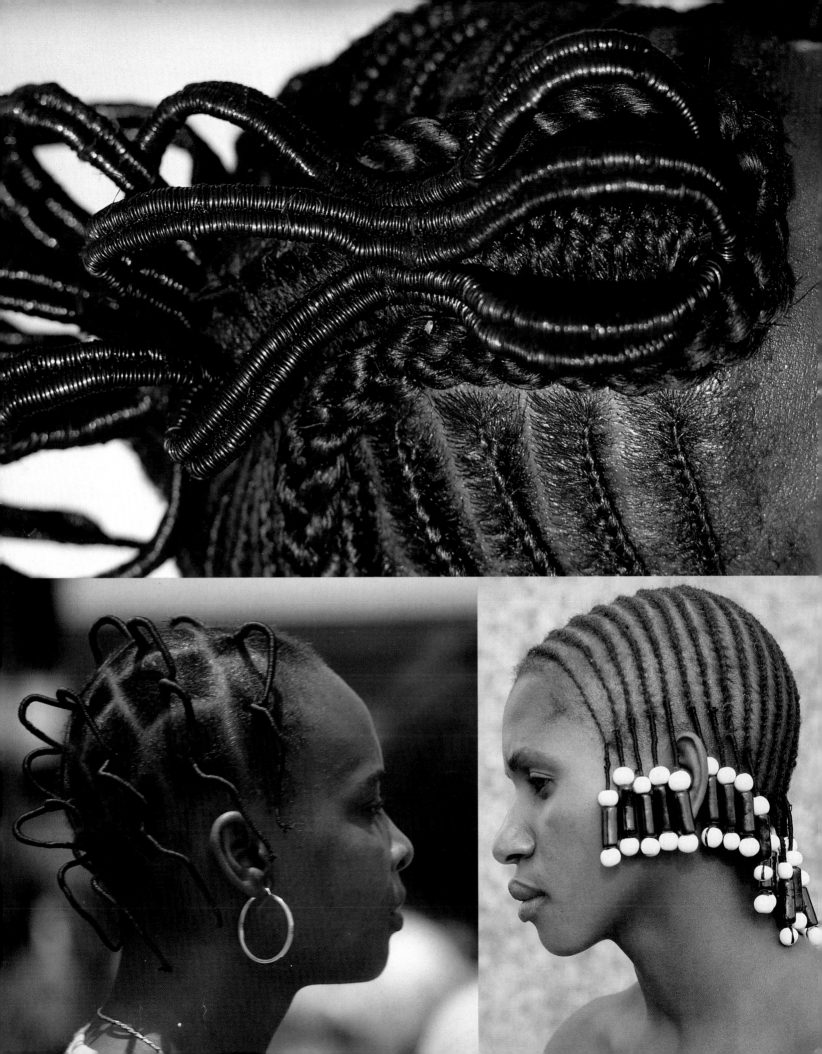

only modest success, though Kate and Jeremy of Haysi Fantayzee succeeded well enough to provoke resentment among true Rastafarians.

To be really authentic, dread-locks require naturally kinky hair which, if left to grow long enough, eventually matts into separate strands. After that, dedicated time-consuming oiling and washing are needed, though no further twisting or plaiting. White followers of the style – deprived of this natural kinkiness – are forced to adopt artificial ways. Some find that false hair twisted into their own growing hair creates a creditable copy but needs hot candle grease dripped on to it to give a good binding effect. This means that washing is impossible and combing out of the question. The only way to get rid of European dread-locks is to cut them off.

African styles are even more difficult to achieve. Some of the most beautiful, such as corn-rowing and plaiting, have been quite successfully attempted by white Caucasians.

But African hair sculpture is a true art. The necessary design skills, the precision and manual dexterity have been handed down for generations. Complex styles take days to produce but they are often so exquisitely becoming it is not surprising that – once discovered – white admirers are often eager to try their hand at copying them.

'Corn-rowing', until recently hidden under wigs by Africans for fear of offending the white establishment, requires plenty of time, plenty of grease and an early decision as to whether to use overhand or underhand technique. Either way, results depend on braiding or plaiting the hair tightly to the scalp and creating intricate patterns in the partings so created. Men's styles are usually more cap-like and flatter to the head than women's styles. Maintaining any style intact involves wrapping a scarf around the head at night and constantly oiling the scalp to keep it in good condition. Pulling the hair so tightly can be painful for the first few days of a new style, and it can also cause dandruff.

Corn-rowing with the addition of attachments demands a more advanced technique. Usually referred to as 'weaving' it requires the help of a hairdresser who will plait and stitch the extra hair into position.

For those graced with longer hair there is also the opportunity for 'threading', a technique borrowed from Nigeria. This involves separating the hair and then winding sections of it with black thread. For sheer fantasy the look is unbeatable, since it offers a three-dimensional style with both a scalp pattern and a design created from threaded strands raised stiffly from the head or nestling in curves on crown or nape of neck. Beads arranged in patterns on the braiding or coloured bobbles at the ends of the threading make attractive elaborations.

What inspired the Skinheads when they made their breakaway from long hair and grease, was quite different. Their concern was not so much beautification or tradition but more assertion of an identity. Descendants of the really hard, mean Mods, Skinheads first appeared in 1964 and literally put the boot in with toe-capped footwear furnished with specially made steel spikes which they went to a lot of trouble to get welded to their boots. Working jeans and braces, donkey jackets and army greens all went well with their cropped hair which no longer required grease. And, said Skinheads triumphantly, cropped hair was useful in scuffles – nothing for the fuzz to get hold of, see? Also, as something of an afterthought, it was easier to keep clean.

For the ignorant and uninitiated, Skins were at pains to explain that stylish Skinhead crops were not crewcuts. Crewcuts, they explained wearily, are close-cut at the sides, and flat on the top. Skinhead haircuts were all-over jobs and you chose your length of stubble and told the barber to get on with it, or else. It was all very time-consuming and expensive, but Skins were devotedly fussy about the crucial length of their crops. Enlightened barbers had four lengths of cut on offer, controlled by a clip-on guard on their electric razor. Number 1 was the shortest cut and number 4 the longest. For extra style, partings were sometimes shaved into the crop from front to crown – a straight copy of West Indian styles.

Skinhead girls, willing accomplices and useful for smuggling weaponry into football matches (girls couldn't so readily be searched) had quite dramatic style. Some grew their hair long and straight. The rest had No. 2 or No. 3 hair crops with a feathered fringe all round. It gave a strangely appealing waif-like look to the face that went well with the fishnet stockings and mini-skirts.

The Punks were different again. They preferred hedgehog hair, spiky and dangerous-looking. They used Vaseline or KY jelly to make it malleable and then – because they had the advantage of aerosols and hair lacquer – styled and sprayed it into obedience. Sometimes they gave it a touch or two of super-glue to make sure it knew the score. Four-inch spikes, stiffened with Bostik, lost at least one young man his job: at Rolls Royce, he was considered to be a danger to fellow workers' eyes.

The individuality which characterised the Punks found colourful expression in the Mohican style. Shaved to inches above the ears, and with its enormous cox-comb flourish, 'The Mohican' became one of the tourist sights of Britain. In Edinburgh, Gary at Technik who had styled a great many Punks said there were three basic types of Punk. And within each group highly individualistic hairstyles were sought. The 'Intelligents' – who were demonstrating through their hair their feelings about the world – were making a social statement. They designed for themselves unique variations which the hairdresser had to execute and which they were prepared and proud to display day and night.

Not so the pin-striped 'Office' Punks. They came out at night exhibiting a totally different persona. They trod a tricky tightrope leading a Jekyll-and-Hyde existence. For this, they required a retractable creation which could be damped down during the day but could come into its own at night. Getting the length right called for nice judgement. It had to be long enough for dramatic effect at night, yet capable of being sleeked down during the working day.

The third group were more abandoned and employed all manner of materials and substances to construct their headdress. They used anything at hand – food colourings, spray-on paints, coloured powders – to pigment their hair. Their scalp was sufficiently shaved to create a canvas for their striking, often aggressive messages to the world. These, they inscribed with water-colour paints, which they then gelled and dried.

BALD IS BEAUTIFUL

The Masai women of East Africa, in contrast, show just what a powerful image the shaven head can create. They smear their shining scalps with red ochre and animal fat – a perfect foil for their accompanying bracelets, head jewellery, earrings and neck adornments. Only for them does hair seem an irrelevance. In extreme contrast, their warrior husbands flatter the striking appearance of their wives. Their hair is grown long and is painstakingly dressed by fellow countrymen in styles which may take anything from fifteen to twenty hours to complete.

In other contexts, closer to home, the shaven head has more often been the mark of the extremist – except where illness or traditional religious practice has rendered it unavoidable. Yet a surprising number of people have voluntarily adopted it.

The German-born poet, Tara Osrik, astounded her New York friends in the 1920s, by shaving her head quite bare and lacquering her newly-exposed cranium a bright vermilion.

Journalist Molly Parkin, too, had her hair shaved when she was a young art student. The barber was reluctant to do it so she told him she had nits, whereupon 'he finished the job in silence and surgical gloves'. On the way home, feeling somewhat bare about the neck, Ms Parkin popped into Woolworths and bought herself a green dog-collar. When she arrived home her parents screamed.

Pop star Sinead O'Connor had her head shaved as a defiant declaration that she was not to be regarded as a 'sex object'. And when model girl Anna Curtis shaved right up to the crown, her colleagues thought she was committing professional suicide. But she knew what she was doing; she went off to Milan and enjoyed non-stop bookings by modelling men's suits for *L'Uomo*. The singer Grace Jones added even more drama to her tall, imposing presence by shaving the back and sides of her head.

Men might at first sight be expected to be reluctant about shaving their heads – they might be taken for a victim of alopecia. Yet many have been surprisingly venturesome. Telly Savalas who first shaved his head for the role of Pontius Pilate in *The Greatest Story Ever Told*, keeps it like that because it has become a valuable 'trade-mark'. Leigh Bowery, who wears curly false eye-lashes and paints his lips to a letter-box square, shaves his head as a finishing touch. Yul Brynner, famously bald in *The King and I*, put on a wig for *The*

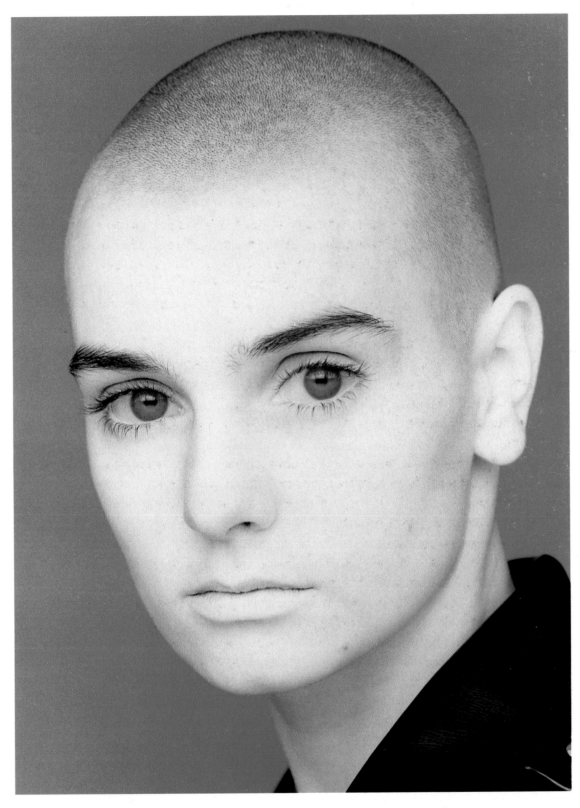

Sinead O'Connor: Defiant shaving of her head has nonetheless enhanced her appeal

Buccaneer – but then returned to the smooth-skulled look by popular demand. Hot Chocolate's rock singer, Erroll Brown quite simply admits, 'A bald head suits my image'.

A fine bald head can clearly have its attractions for the opposite sex. When, after fifteen years, Ray Milland threw away his wig for *Love Story*, they say that matrons became suddenly 'weak at the knees'.

But what of the millions who mourn the loss of their youthful head of hair? The decision to astonish by removing hair voluntarily is one thing – losing it without choice is quite another. Most men's reaction is sadness tempered with resignation, or an avowed determination to conceal the loss by some means or other. Hopes of restoration may have been eternal – but alas, they have invariably been dashed. The secret of giving back to hair its ability to regenerate has eluded scientists, trichologists and beauticians for thousands of years.

RESTORATION?

There have been recipes for restoring hair ever since the first man noticed he was losing it.

In ancient Egypt, the heel of an Abyssinian greyhound mixed with date blossoms and asses' hooves boiled in oil was guaranteed to do the trick. Hippocrates, 'Father of Medicine', recommended to the Greeks poultices containing pigeons' droppings, cumin and nettles. In the sixteenth century, one frantic suggestion was to massage the scalp with a mixture of burnt male faeces and the ashes of a hedgehog.

Baldness is no respecter of persons. The noble Julius Caesar clung to his laurel wreath because it hid his lack of hair. Napoleon mourned the early loss of his hair: it would at least have given him some extra height. Women who begin to go thin on top are even more distraught. Elizabeth I, whose maltreated hair became thin very early, relied on a pomade made from apples and puppy-dog fat. But by the time she had reached her thirties she had lost the struggle and most of her hair had fallen out. Diane de Poitiers, mistress of Henri II of France, refused to give up. As her hair became noticeably thinner, she used a liquor made up specially for her by the alchemist Paracelsus; it contained, as gossip had it, the blood of a murdered, new-born baby.

Modern science has produced some powerful remedies. Some of these mimic the body's natural substances such as its hormones. Hair lotions have been produced containing oestrogen, in an attempt to counteract the male hormone which triggers baldness. Unfortunately, side-effects were produced such as gynecomastia, the growth of breasts and darkening of the areola in males. The extreme sensitivity of the male body to the female hormone was demonstrated when a seventy-year-old male began to develop breasts following contact with the oestrogen cream which his wife was using for vaginitis.

Today, baldness in varying degrees affects about 50% of the male population.

Hormonal disturbance, excessive dandruff or eczema, certain drugs – particularly those used in the treatment of cancer – as well as anxiety and stress can all be contributory causes. The major culprit, however, is the inherited baldness gene which can run relentlessly through generations of families. Men are especially unfortunate. All it takes is one set of genes and they will inherit a tendency to hair loss. And when that particular gene is present, a man's production of sex hormones simply adds further to the likelihood of hair loss.

It's a Catch 22 situation for a man if, by using drugs for example, he attempts to reduce his testosterone level, he does so at his peril: loss of libido may follow. There is only one certain cure which would safeguard the future of a young male member of a family known to be carrying the gene, and which would, at the same time, considerably reduce the possibility of any later dynastic baldness: castration.

Women are more fortunate. They need two genes – one from each parent – before they are affected: and then it will only be active after the menopause when their production of female hormones is reduced. Even this can be remedied by Hormone Replacement Therapy.

But we live in an age of constant discovery. There is now, at long last, hope for at least some who have lost their hair. The most promising hair restorer yet – neatly named 'Regaine' – became available in 1988 on private prescription. Made by the drug company Upjohn, its major ingredient is minoxidil, a substance which can be found naturally in rat's urine. Its discovery had about it more than a touch of serendipity. A United States heart doctor, who was prescribing it to lower blood pressure, noticed that the balding heads of his patients were sprouting anew with springtimes of fresh hair growth. Naturally, the word got about and use of minoxidil specifically for hair regeneration began, albeit under cover. Experts are still hotly debating the extent of its usefulness. Most reckon that the chance of promoting hair growth by using this drug is no more than 50% – younger men having a better chance of recovery than older men. Women have used it too, with some success.

But even in the world of miracle cures, things do not stand still. Del De Laronde-Wilton, an economist who founded a 'National Hair Clinic' in October 1987, has already overtaken and updated the product 'Regaine'. Impressed by the number of desperate men who were appealing to him for help – including one who was so terrified of losing more hair that he hadn't washed his hair with shampoo for eighteen months – he tried adding a small amount of retinoic acid to the Regaine/minoxidil formula. Retinoic acid – used for years in the treatment of juvenile acne – has the effect of abrading the skin so that minoxidil may be absorbed by the scalp more readily.

Arthur Knight, consultant dermatologist at the University Hospital of Wales, summed up the minoxidil discovery: 'It is not a charlatan treatment. If used on people with male pattern balding, minoxidil does appear to slow down the process quite substantially and cause some re-growth. The problem is that the effects wear off, so you have to keep using it indefinitely.'

So here is a dilemma for modern men just as tricky as that which has beset women ever since expensive female rejuvenation treatments became available. The question is, will men be willing to commit themselves to a lifetime of routine treatment? Has anyone enquired about the implications for their blood pressure? Are they prepared to spend approximately £30 to £50 a month to keep their hair on?

There might just be another possible solution: oxygen. The chief of surgery and director of research at the United States Naval Hospital in Long Beach, California, Dr George Hurt, treats divers for 'the bends' by getting them to breathe pure oxygen in a pressure chamber. Now, his divers are reporting that their thinning hair is growing again. Better than that – they have found that they are more virile. But this double-bonus treatment is still being investigated.

TRANSPLANTATION

In the late 1970s Elton John went to France for a hair transplant. Nevertheless he is rarely seen in public without his hat, which has become his 'trade-mark'.

Hair transplanting, if successful, can cunningly – and more equably – rearrange the remaining hair still growing, either by swinging round a strip of scalp from the hairy part of the head and 're-turfing' a bald patch, or by punch-grafting: making holes in the scalp and then lifting a modest number of hairs – say ten – along with an area of skin, and replanting this in the holes. The leader of a pop group in Wales described his operation as 'excruciatingly painful'. But he feels committed to undergo more, if only to get rid of what forthright critics have called his 'colander look'.

Surgeons warn that the operation is not always successful. A scar may be left and this may become hard and keloidal. Trouble can arise if too many hairs are taken at one time.

One man blamed his balding head on his wife's leaving him for another man. In despair, he underwent an ambitious – quite excessive – transplant of no less than 600 grafts – and woke up to find his pillow saturated with blood.

'The majority of implantees have local or systemic infections, either of which may be life threatening,' according to *The Journal of the American Medical Association*. There have been so many horrifying examples of transplant disasters: they describe the typical patient as having a scalp that resembles a piece of stinking red meat with pus pouring out.

It is curious that the painful and difficult technique has been so much explored by men and so little by women. For men, after all, baldness is a clear masculine signal; for women it is a tragedy.

SUPPLEMENTATION

There is yet another possible solution – which is to thicken up any existing hair with extra real or artificial hair. But this has to be done in good time. Men who have already lost their hair cannot bind or twist additional hair to their scalp if there is no stubble left to anchor it to. Wigs and toupees remain for them the only other solution.

Women are again more fortunate. They usually manage to retain some hair, however frail and thin it may become. And this they can discreetly add to with chignons and swatches for use during the daytime.

For the really grand occasion, more substantial supplementations may be employed, something which the ladies of other lands have often exploited to striking effect. The Sango women of the Congo have no hesitation in removing the hair of the dead – or hair taken from prisoners – and adding it to their own long hair as well as palm fibres painted black. The great disadvantage is that such coiffures – which take many weeks to complete – are expected to last, sometimes for months, before dismantling, during which time, naturally enough, they lose more than a little of their pristine freshness.

Western women for over a hundred years accepted this sanitary disability without – as it were – turning a hair. It was all just part of the price of beauty. Not only did seventeenth- and eighteenth-century ladies lose sleep in an effort to keep their towering heads of hair intact. They caused carriage seats to be lowered and door-posts to be raised, all to accommodate the ornate coiffures.

'They press against the temples, prevent the circulation of the blood and cause abscesses. Some die in consequence.' Such were the effects of metal wires used in the extravagant headdresses of the times and described in a letter dated 1685 from Madame de Sévigné to her daughter.

The fashion for tall heads was taken up by French and English women alike. Coiffures climbed as much as two feet high, heavily padded, decorated and tethered by a multitude of lace ribbons, with long strands of hair mounted bravely on tall, brass wires.

And there were other problems. Ladies were so top heavy that they were forced to kneel in their carriages. The *Gentleman's Magazine* of 1777 reported that the seats of coaches were sunk almost to the bottom of the carriage, the ladies sitting with their knees pushed into the pits of their stomachs. Even so they were compelled to travel bending forward to avoid touching the roof.

A great deal of time and patience was needed to build up these hairstyles. First there was the elaborate, underlying framework and the padding (often made from greased wool and horsehair). Then the natural hair was built up over this and plastered into place with a sticky concoction of paste, followed by further supplements of false hair. Then came the ornaments. These might take the form of vegetables, fruits, feathers, and even baskets of flowers. Sometimes the flowers were provided with sustaining water in bottles and vases

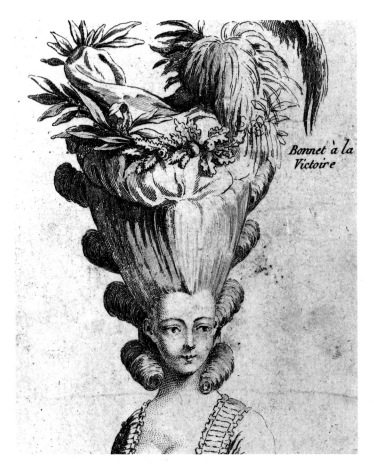

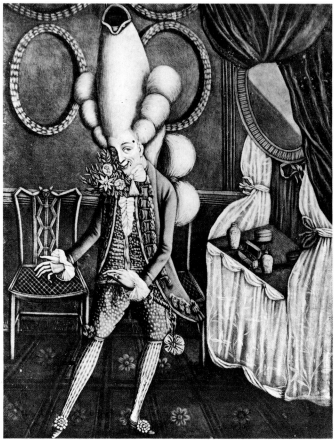

L E F T : Seventeenth- and eighteenth-century ladies had to sleep sitting up in order to keep their towering heads of hair intact

R I G H T : Eighteenth-century men were just as vain as women, as this French caricature of a Macaroni shows

cunningly hidden within the hair. To walk without spillage meant that the ladies' movements were necessarily stiff and awkward as they manoeuvred their water-laden heads around corners and under arches.

There was, of course, the awkward question of going to bed. Many ladies, having spent half a day with a hairdresser 'making a head' and not wishing prematurely to spoil it, found it simpler not to go to bed at all. Instead, they sat up, dozing the night away in chairs, and carefully preserving every contrived foot of their splendid headpieces.

Fire was a continual hazard to the lady who was determined to walk tall. Rooms were decorated with chandeliers holding dozens of candles and it was not unusual for madam to light up all too suddenly, in mid-sentence.

Combing was out of the question, in view of the elaborate styling of the hair. As for washing it, this was strictly a twice-yearly event. In fact, when Lord Chesterfield heard that the ladies of Bath were wearing their hair, 'three or four storeys high' he was heard to growl, 'Yes, and I believe every storey is inhabited like the loding [lodging] houses here, for I observe a great deal of scratching.'

There were other troubles too. The constant larding of the hair attracted mice, and nests with whole families of them were frequently found in a woman's hair. It says much for the ladies' ingenuity and spirit that they remained undaunted; they tackled the problem by spreading a yard or two of protective mesh over their rancid heads at night. Larded, rancid and covered in mesh, bearing upon their loved ones with possibly a rodent or two for company, they could hardly have made enticing bedmates. As the *London Magazine* of 1768 put it:

. . . I went the other morning to make a visit to an elderly aunt of mine when I found her tendering her head to the ingenious Mr. Gilchrist, who had lately obliged the public with a most excellent essay upon hair. He asked her how long it was since her head had been opened or repaired. She replied not above nine weeks. To which he replied that was as long as a head could well go in the summer, and that therefore it was proper to deliver it now for he confessed that it began to be a little 'hazarde'.

When Mr. Gilchrist opened my aunt's head, as he called it, . . . I observed swarms of animalculaes running about in the utmost consternation and in different directions upon which I put my chair a little further away from the table and asked the operator whether that numerous swarm did not from time to time send out colonies to other parts of the body? He assured me that they could not; for that quantity of powder and pomatum formed a glutinous matter, which lime, like twigs to birds, caught and clogged the little natives and prevented their migration.

In old Japan several assistants were commonly needed to wash, pomade and plait a lady's hair to provide her with a similar elaborate coiffure. And the fashion dies hard. Even at the beginning of the twentieth century, five hours or more were willingly being spent by dedicated teams, in the building up of a lady's coiffure. Modern Geisha girls who retain the traditional, elaborately coiled hairstyles, still spend many hours in its preparation and keep it intact by sleeping on a specially fashioned head-rest.

9. SMALL IS BEAUTIFUL: THE FEET

There has never been a time when it was fashionable for a lady to have big feet. Indeed, this is one of the rare fixtures in the restless history of female beauty. Only the Turks have ever been prepared to value large feet in women and then only because they associate high fertility with them.

LOTUSES OF GOLD, SILVER AND IRON

The Chinese ridiculed and outlawed the big female foot but went even further. They set about making it smaller and smaller by compressing it more and more until it measured a mere three inches. And for a thousand years, Chinese daughters wept.

How the idea arose of binding the foot to reduce it to a mere three inches remains a mystery. One story from India may provide a hint: it tells of a beautiful human child born to a roe-deer – perfect in every way save that the little girl had the feet of a deer. Wherever she trod she left impressions in the ground which resembled the marks of the revered lotus flower. And to the Eastern mind the lotus is the embodiment of all that is romantic, beautiful and blessed.

Perhaps the Chinese concubines re-enacted in their dancing this story of the deer-child with the tiny lotus-tread. Certainly, a style of dancing involving just a little foot-binding had become popular by the time of the T'ang dynasty between the tenth and eleventh centuries. Ironically, therefore, it may have been through dancing that the bound foot was introduced to China. By the time of the Sung dynasty in the twelfth century, feminine liberty and intellectual freedom were being increasingly frowned on. The ideal woman was docile, not argumentative. She must therefore never be in a position to make comparisons between her own and others' menfolk; instead, she should be confined to the boudoir, and here, with her horizons clipped, and her knowledge of other men limited, she would be incapable of any form of conjugal infidelity.

The bound foot, already popular among the dancing girls, fitted neatly into this new climate of masculine domination. What better way of restraining a woman's movements and her adventurous spirit than by binding her feet?

Strangely, these women do not appear to have been unduly worried by their second-class citizenship, or even their restricted movement. What they were much more concerned about was the achievement of small feet which would at one stroke qualify them as beautiful, fashionable and distinctly upper-class. Only peasant women had large feet; a lady of refinement should always have small feet. And there was yet another bonus. Such a lady – as was later to become clear – would also be more sexually attractive. Her 'golden lotuses' would bring added pleasure to her husband and so fulfil woman's obvious and most important duty, that of pleasing a man.

Soon it was realised that though adult feet could be reduced with a certain amount of success, children's feet would yield to pressure in a much more rapid and effective way.

Chinese mothers did not hesitate. Determined that their daughters should not be left behind in the struggle for the three-inch 'golden lotus' which would ensure a prosperous marriage, they conscientiously rushed with needles, binding cloths and ruthless determination to bend their children's toes during those tender years when the infant feet were at their most vulnerable. Children had little choice in the matter. Most of them, with extraordinary stoicism, accepted their mother's conviction that footbinding was essential.

As one woman later explained: 'The majority of girls had their feet bound whether they liked it or not. However, when the mother started the binding, the girl would cry out with pain and wish to discontinue. If the girls had a chance, they would secretly undo the bindings. Sometimes, because of the tightness of the binding, the girl's feet became swollen and the skin turned a bluish colour. Mothers did not let their daughters untie the bindings, because they wanted them to look like members of rich families. In order to prevent unbinding, they therefore tied their hands to a pole. In this way they could not undo the binding.'

One woman, whose feet had been bound when she was nine, insisted that it was all worth while.

'Mother was very strict. My foot felt very painful at the start. The heel of my foot became odoriferous and deteriorated. Because of the pain in my foot, my whole body became emaciated. My face colour changed and I couldn't sleep at night, frightening my mother. When I saw how pretty the tiny feet of others were, I liked that very much. My cousin told me that no one wanted to marry a woman with big feet'.

Binding began at about five years of age, the object being to bring the sole and heel as close together as was physically possible. A bandage about two inches wide and ten feet long was placed with one end on the inside of the instep, and then carried over the little toes so as to force the toes in and under and back towards the sole. Then the bandage would be wrapped around the heel with such force that heel and toes were drawn closer together.

The child suffered dreadfully. Soon the foot would become putrescent; portions of flesh would often come away from the sole and toes would drop off, causing intense pain. The only hope of relief was that after two years or so the feet might become mercifully dead and painless. But this did not always happen.

Ritual and ceremony surrounded the commencement of binding. This was an important moment in a girl's life: an auspicious day had to be chosen when moon, and other celestial auguries were favourable. Congratulatory visits from relatives were made to houses where foot-binding was about to start, the object being to signal to the mother that her intentions were honourable, correct, and understood by all to be in the best interests of the child.

The girls themselves had always been told that they could expect to suffer twice for beauty in their lives, first when they had their ears pierced, and then when they had their feet bound.

The suffering was intense: little girls of seven years old, with newly-bound feet felt they were on fire and could not sleep. When they ate fish or freshly killed meat their feet would swell and the pus would drip. But mothers forced their daughters to walk, and often criticised them for placing too much pressure on the heel. Every two weeks new shoes were brought to the child – each new pair one-fifth of an inch smaller.

For two years or so this appalling ritual went on. It was a time of unbelievable agony when little sisters would weep together, dreading the moment of exercise and the arrival of ever smaller shoes.

For the Chinese woman, her feet became the great preoccupation of her life. Everywhere the 'golden lotus' was a talking-point among the ladies – especially for those with daughters approaching foot-binding age. And inevitably, advisers and experts would pontificate on the attributes of the perfect foot. Lyrical descriptions abounded, imaginations soared in the seeking out of evocative titles. Thus the compressed hoof might be romantically dubbed 'Divine Quality' or 'Seductive Attitude'. Size, of course, was the main consideration: a foot might be a lotus of 'gold' (three inches), 'silver' (four inches) or 'iron' (four inches or more).

But always, the final arbiters of quality were men. And by all accounts they were generous in their praise. The tiny foot was well worth striving for, they said, for it was such an exquisite plaything. Indeed, the mere glimpse of a Chinese lady binding the 'golden lotus' could cause a man to groan with passion:

> Oh! how tiny they are
> Like broken winter bamboo shoots
> And like dumplings in May.

What greater encouragement could a woman have?

Eventually, the tiny foot became so treasured that it developed into a mysterious object of devotion, a kind of private shrine to be concealed at all times from the lewd gaze of others. So a woman was never allowed to display her feet. She invariably unwrapped her foot-bindings in private and was never seen without her shoes, even in bed. And since the shoes lived in such enviable intimacy with the feet, they too became objects of devotion. Women were taught to make their own shoes, often lavishing a great deal of time and effort on them. Colour was most important: red and green were popular, but over many centuries of foot-binding, red was always the favourite. Red shoes signalled the exciting woman. Love under the bedclothes with the flash of a red silk shoe – glimpsed against the gleaming ivory of a woman's skin – was one of the great fantasies of amorous play. Indeed, a woman's little red night shoes were often pitted with toothmarks, ample proof that they had been seized in moments of high passion and smothered with the kisses and bites of her excited partner.

The shoes were stored in a special drawer in the bedroom, and since there was always the possibility they might be nibbled by ardent lovers they were kept fragrant by the presence of sachets of perfume tucked inside them.

Respectable ladies kept their feet to themselves and were deeply ashamed if they were accidentally touched, especially by the vulgar or low-born. It was by no means unknown for a desperate Chinese gentleman to crawl on all fours through the feet of a crowd to reach out and touch a tiny foot which had momentarily caused him to lose his reason. The results could be disastrous: one girl, furtively stroked in this way by a foot frotteur, took to her bed and died of shame. Illicit love-making addressed to forbidden shoes often took place, and profane acts with the stolen shoes of a loved one were sometimes performed by rejected lovers, who then returned the soiled and abused shoes as an insult. This ancient form of 'heavy breathing' caused ladies great distress and feelings of insult.

There were rules for the amorous about how to hold the tiny foot. For purist gentlemen, a manual on love play was available for consultation. Such a book never failed to describe the various techniques for grasping the precious lotus in ultimate erotic passion.

Exciting bodily changes in the woman were believed to take place following foot-binding. For example, she was said to develop exceptionally voluptuous hips and powerful thighs – a direct result of placing so much weight on her thighs and hips. Even more visually alluring was the tense, cringing posture she had to adopt while trying to keep the weight off her feet when walking. And all of this had such an effect on her more intimate anatomy that she was believed to acquire the permanent muscular tone of a virgin – a great boon in athletic love-making.

Pheromones were active too, the tiny foot having a delightful arousal odour superior to that emanating from armpits, legs and other glandular sources. Tasting the foot was a special treat. One Nanking official declared that, above all else, he enjoyed washing, smelling and tasting his concubine's small feet; licking them during washing was, he said, 'like eating steamed dumplings in pure water'.

Husbands were unanimous in their conviction that the tiny-footed woman made the best bedmate. Even apart from love-making, if she placed herself against you when you slept, you did not feel a heavy weight, and this was most agreeable. A large-footed woman moving under the bedcovers was less desirable – she could cause an annoying draught of cold air. With so much in its favour, it seemed inconceivable that foot-binding in China would ever end.

Men, too, occasionally had their feet bound. This was because in the fifteenth century so much store was placed on the pronouncements and predictions of astrologers. Sometimes the families of young boys were told that the future of this son of theirs looked dark – so dark and inauspicious in fact that it would be better if they reared the boy as a girl. So the boy's feet were bound; he was dressed in feminine clothes, and thereafter passed off as a female. If an offer of marriage came his way, the young man in bride's clothing might wait until the groom had provided the customary dowry: and then – quite frequently – he would make off with it.

A modern kind of foot-binding was practised too, by men in Tientsin, in about 1900. They wrapped their feet up firmly with cloth and compressed them with hard, tight socks – all so that they could wear the narrow brocade shoes which were all the rage.

By this time, however, the days of female foot-binding were numbered. In 1928, the Ministry of Domestic Affairs formally prohibited the practice, threatening any recalcitrant foot-binders with substantial fines. This placed women in a cruelly difficult position because unbinding the feet was almost as painful as binding them. Caught in this conflict of changing standards they had no choice but to endure pain twice over. With broken bones and swollen insteps they stumbled and fell in their efforts to walk.

And watching them, Chinese men had heavy hearts. They had lost their golden-lotus playmates. There would be no more tiny-footed women, no more girls with red satin shoes on their three-inch feet, no more docile girls who had big thighs, who could not run away and who – when they turned over in bed – did not create a draught.

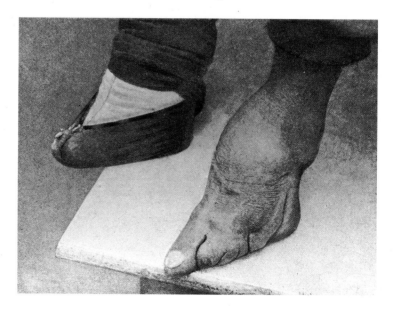

OPPOSITE: A Chinese beauty and (ABOVE) the appealing Chinese foot

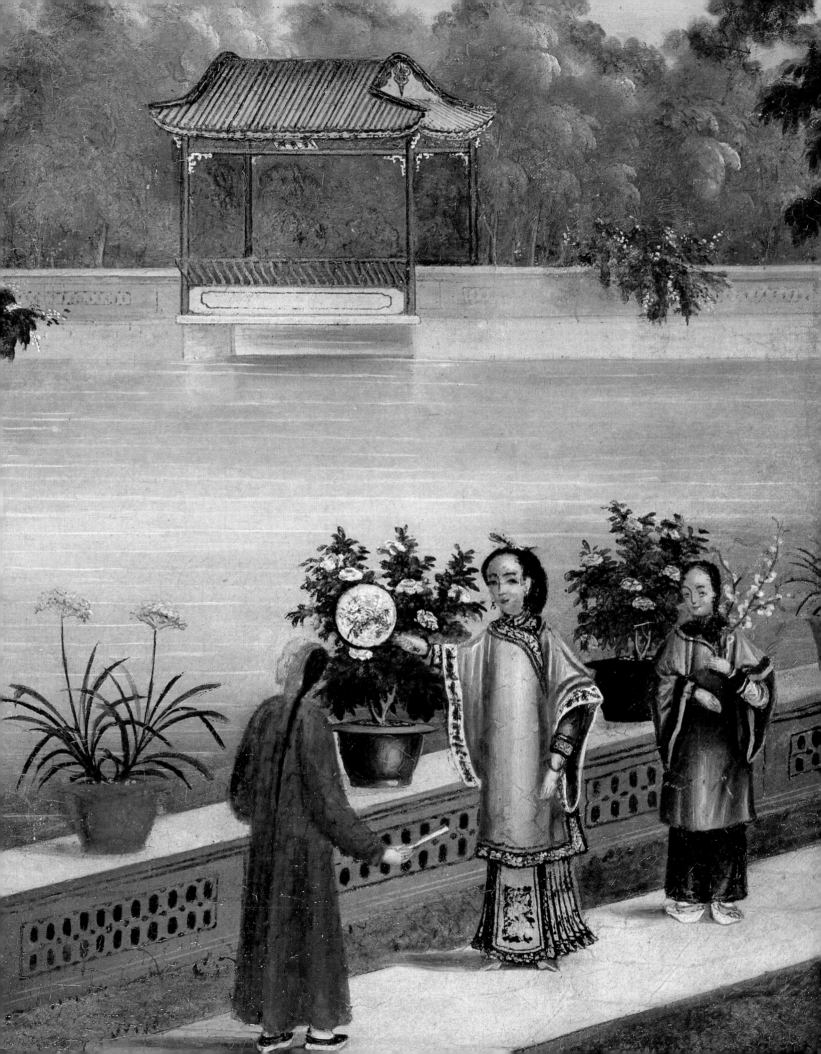

THE FOOT MUST FIT THE FASHION

To accommodate her feet in the narrowest of winkle-picker court shoes, model girl Barbara Goalen had both her little toes amputated. Chiropodists will find nothing surprising about that; *The Journal of Podiatry* has already pointed out that whenever there is a resurgence of shoes with pointed toes there is an increase in the demand for foot surgery.

'You must suffer if you want to be beautiful . . . better to lose a toe than a Queen's throne', says a Danish version of *Cinderella*. The story has its parallels today: fashion is the glass slipper which decides shape and style – and women's feet must obediently fit the fashion.

Not surprising then that more than half the adults in the UK have something wrong with their feet. Women deform their feet not only with poor footwear but also with nylon tights which cause their toes to hump and curl under. But most astonishing, as one chiropodist has pointed out, 'more than half of those who think that their shoes are the cause of their problems say they wear them, knowingly, because of fashion'.

The problems start early. As chiropodist Brian Berry points out, the woolly bootees and stretch-suits worn by babies almost always shrink; the baby, on the other hand, grows, but can for a time continue to wear the same suit. He recommends that mothers cut off the toe-tops of bootees and stretch-suits as baby feet become bigger.

But there is little to be gained by appealing to shoemakers to ignore those fashions which demand shapes so out of tune with the human foot. And little point in asking them to create instead comfortable, sensible shoes. Only when her feet have been battered into the need for orthopaedic footwear will a woman turn to shoes which offer comfort before style. So shoemakers stick to their lasts for purely commercial reasons, and who can blame them? The pity of it is, their lasts are shaped by fashion.

Shoes are big business and for good reason: they give the final touch to dress, coat or suit. Women – and quite a lot of men – love them. Actress Cher is especially fond of her feet and boasts more than three hundred pairs of shoes, all in 'sexy styles'. Singer Diana Ross says, 'I've got beautiful legs and I want to show them off with beautiful shoes'. Joan Fontaine, Dietrich, Joan Crawford have all owned more than a hundred pairs of shoes at a time.

Jayne Mansfield once owned two hundred pairs. Even the large-footed Garbo once bought seventy pairs of Ferragamo's shoes at one visit. The Empress Josephine, wife of Napoleon, had a collection of five hundred pairs, some so fragile they could only be worn while she remained seated. And Marie Antoinette had so many hundreds of pairs she had to index them methodically in an impressive record book. Only one woman seems to have eclipsed her – Mrs Marcos, wife of the deposed President of the Philippines – whose collection ran into thousands.

Whether shoes are necessary at all depends on habitat and environment. Most footwear experts recommend that in the interests of health, the ideal would be to wear no shoes at all. The Aborigines of Australia and millions of both Asian and American Indians wander their native lands without protection – and without foot problems. Yoga enthusiasts and foot reflexologists are unanimous in their advice: 'Go without shoes around the house whenever you can.'

Yet these are voices crying in the wilderness. For centuries, compression and contortion of the foot, together with the idea of walking daintily, taking only tiny steps, has held a unique fascination for both Western and Oriental women. In old Palestine, girls managed to achieve a mincing gait by attaching slave chains to their feet, the shorter the chain, the tinier – and therefore more elegant – the step. The cult ankle-chains which appeared on boots for 'Punk chicks' in the 1970s did not directly restrict movement, but the uncomfortable, high-heeled, pointed-toe shape of the boot itself made walking difficult and a short-stepped shuffle was often the result. It was not just a sense of self-importance and defiance among their owners which gave these boots the label 'strutters'.

The compulsion to walk with difficulty has been satisfied in completely different and sometimes amazing ways. In the fourteenth century, slippers with long pointed toes were fashionable – the higher the rank the longer the toe. In order to be able to walk at all, Anne of Bohemia (1366–99) fastened the points of her shoes above her calves with long, golden chains. Other aristocratic ladies attached silver bells to the points of their shoes before tying them to their knees – the 'bells on her toes' of the old nursery rhyme.

To have small, narrow feet was the mark of the aristocrat in the seventeenth and eighteenth centuries. So high-born European ladies bound their feet at night with strips of waxed linen.

Even in the twentieth century, there is a feeling – not too far below the surface – that tightly-clad legs and tiny feet are the mark, not only of high fashion and femininity, but also of high breeding. In the late 1920s, an over-enthusiastic teacher at an expensive finishing school for girls in the States was discovered to be zealously instructing her young charges to bind their feet at night using linen tapes. 'Anyone knows,' she said at her subsequent court case, 'that every well-bred gentleman considers this a mark of good breeding in a woman.'

Victorian women were doubly unfortunate in the matter of footwear. In earlier centuries shoes had been made to measure but in the 1820s machines for making shoes were invented. Unhappily, they created shapes which were in no way connected with the true outlines of the foot. Also, the fashion at the time was for narrow, straight shoes with little difference between the toe-end and the heel-end. Feet were expected to accommodate to the shoe, not the other way round. Worse still, even when a few comfortable impressions had been made, fashion-conscious Victorian ladies transferred the 'left' shoe to the right foot so that both shoes might remain 'nice and straight'. In the United States of America

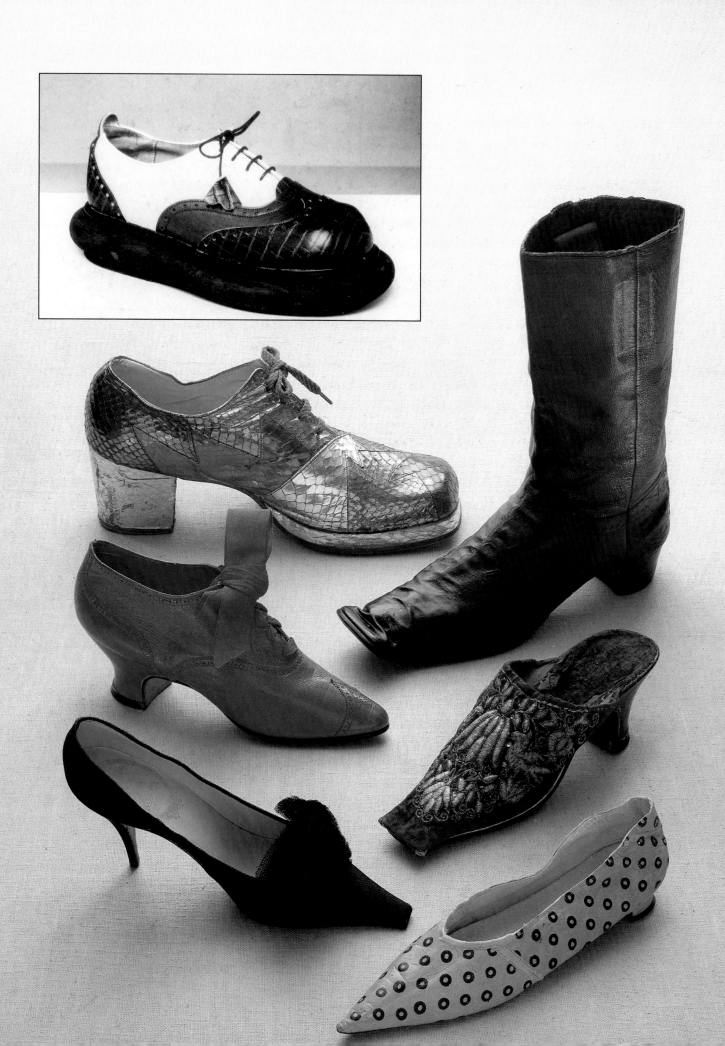

too, at the beginning of the nineteenth century, there were no lefts and rights. People preferred the symmetrical look of straight shoes, and were prepared to wear their shoes on either foot, to keep them so.

But the long-term damage caused to the foot by the wearing of ill-fitting shoes may be devastating, and permanent. Victorian feet were afflicted with ingrown toe nails and painful joints – all of which were taken for granted. It was expected that feet would hurt. Today's feet are no better. Bunion joints and humped toes, together with regular crops of corns and calluses often drive modern women into wearing – without any choice – exactly those non-flattering shoes they have hitherto rejected. One shoe sufferer in the United States had already endured so many years of discomfort that she could only rejoice in the eventual discovery of 'sensible' shoes. In a letter to a shoe store she was incoherent with gratitude: 'For ten years my feet hurt me. The last couple of years my feet have been so tender and sore I couldn't even sleep with my husband. After wearing your comfort shoes for only two months I now find I can sleep with anyone.'

Once upon a time boots were practical. They might be wellington boots, riding boots or motorbike boots. Or traditional army boots. But in the early Sixties, boots suddenly became fashion currency. The trend began in the late 1950s in coffee-bars and cellars where young men who were sharp dressers wore Italian-styled shoes, with pointed toes and elastic sides instead of laces. But this new style was soon transmuted into a high-sided boot with a Cuban heel, dignified by the title 'Beat' boot. In Liverpool, they were worn by a group of music-makers whose sound became so popular that very soon the youth of the world wanted not only to sound like them . . . but to look like them. 'Beat' boots were part of the look. But from now on, they became known as 'Beatle boots'.

These 'Beatle Boots' of the Sixties started a craze which remained popular through the Seventies and into the Eighties. Knee-length cowboy-boots with fancy stitching, strolled the corrals of the High Street – bike boots with buckles appeared on the dance floor – grounded aviators made love in pilot boots. There were boots with rocker platforms, commando boots and of course, the famous Doc Marten steel-cap 'bovver boots'. By the early 1970s Elton John, The Tubes and other pop stars were making stages quiver as they stomped around in platform-soles with heels more than six inches high. Punk purists added safety-pin buckles. Women joined in the boot boom. For 'Punk sisters' – those 'chicks who don't give a damn' – boots were graphically named. There were 'Bloody Mary's' and 'Trouble Makers', in patent leather and in colours appropriately 'Razor Red', 'Bondage Black', and 'Slash Yellow'. Quick off the mark, Mary Quant had already liaised with the stark, 'space-age' clothes of Courrèges and introduced stylish boots for other fashion-conscious women. Fashion model Twiggy who says she has never liked her legs because they are too thin took to them right away. Boots remain her greatest passion – which is perhaps why she owns about two hundred pairs. The leather industry rejoiced as

O P P O S I T E : Fashion has rarely produced either sensible or comfortable shoes. *Clockwise*: Wellington boot, English, 1820s; mule, English, 1790s; kid shoe, English, 1790s; satin shoe, French, 1954; laced shoe, English, c. 1900; platform shoe by Terry de Havilland, 1972. *Inset*: Hover shoes by Red or Dead, 1989 more and more women discovered that they liked the look of their hide-bound legs and feet. Nancy Sinatra and Honor Blackman supplied the finishing touches and made boots immortal.

But by the 1970s, problems of a medical kind had begun to emerge. Dr Paul H. Steel sounded the alarm in *The Journal of the American Medical Association* in 1971. He was worried by the increasing incidence of 'boot leg phlebitis' caused by the wearing of leg-length boots which restricted the circulation and led to blood clots. His warnings were totally ignored.

EROTIC FEET – EROTIC SHOES

As well as being a mark of good breeding, the foot has gained a reputation as a love object. Such a reputation, involving erotic and potentially sinful powers, has not gone unnoticed by the Church. In the third century, St Clement of Alexandria commanded women not to reveal their toes in public. Indeed, the whole purpose of a shoe in the eyes of the Church was to bring propriety to the foot and so remove temptation and lusting from men's hearts.

In seventeenth-century Spain, a lady's foot was considered a most personal part of her anatomy and there was a great hullabaloo when someone suggested that long skirts be raised just sufficiently to avoid soiled hemlines. Spaniards heatedly declared they would rather see their daughters dead than allow them to reveal their feet to the eyes of other men. In some parts of the USA, as recently as the early twentieth century, the selling of a button-boot was so fraught with problems that the salesman's job might be at risk. If he accidentally raised a skirt above the shinline, or worse, touched a woman's ankle, he ran the risk of being fired on the spot.

There was much the same regard for the intimacy of the foot in Britain in the time of Victoria. Women's feet were not supposed to show under their crinolines. But if they did, they might only be tolerated and excused if they were small. Ambitious mothers jammed their daughters' feet into the smallest possible footwear just as their Chinese counterparts had been doing for centuries.

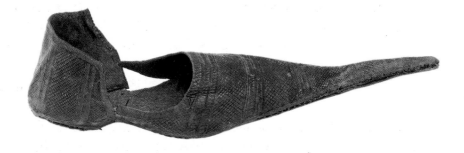

The poulaine – eventually condemned for its erotic overtones

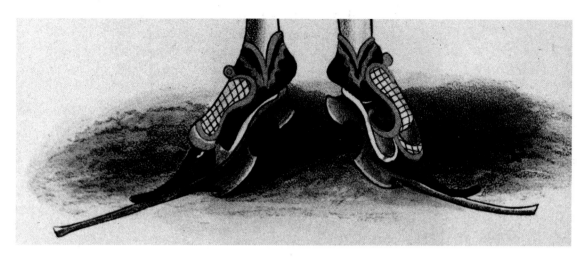

Psychologists have tried to explain the powerful imagery of the foot. Both Jung and Freud declared that dreams which involve shoes being forcefully removed indicated a fear of castration. Karl A. Menninger has pointed out that all nations in legend and literature associate sexual activity with the foot. He also believes that the act of uncovering another's foot is a declaration of sexual possession. Rudofsky, in *The Unfashionable Human Body*, asserts that 'feet' is frequently a euphemism for 'genitalia'.

In the Middle Ages men began to recognise the sexual invitation they might offer through their shoes. And very 'pointed' it was too. A long shoe, which tapered to an arrow-like end became universally popular, enjoyed a scandalous 300-year-run, and was called the Poulaine. It was worn first by Count Fulk of Anjou simply to give ease to an ingrown toe-nail, but the implications of its size and shape were impossible to avoid especially when, as it grew longer – sometimes to fourteen inches or more – it was stuffed to keep it erect and was blatantly coloured at its end. Beneath the dinner table a male poulaine was capable of raising the skirt of the female opposite and – depending on her reception and adventurous spirit – could go on an infamous voyage of exploration. This probing pedic dildo was upsetting to digestion, to say the least, and there were many official and unofficial attempts to stamp it out altogether.

Perhaps in the interests of setting an example to students – thirteenth-century professors at the University of Paris were singled out and forbidden to wear them. All sorts of reasons for not wearing them were invented: even the Black Plague was blamed on the poulaine and men were begged to heed the terrible warning. The Church said that poulaines hampered the devout when kneeling at their prayers. But men continued to sport them.

Eventually a peculiar compromise was reached. The thrust of the shoe was limited to six inches for commoners, up to twenty-four inches for the aristocracy and no restrictions whatsoever for kings and princes. These bewildering equations lasted until 1463 when England's Edward IV literally put his foot down and made a two-inch probe the law for

A B O V E : Fifteenth-century poulaine with protective wooden sole everyone. Whereupon the fire went out of the fashion – the 300-year-reign of this 'cock-of-the-walk' ended – and men had to wait a few years longer before the poulaine's titillating charms could be replaced by the equally flamboyant cod-piece.

The abundant modern literature on sex is full of accounts of strange erotic practices involving the feet. One American woman was found massaging her feet with the nozzle of the Hoover; it was not just a divertingly ticklish business but – so we are told – a richly sensuous experience. Unfortunately, in her case there were complications. She was said to be too exhausted after her vac. trips to be bothered with her husband.

Even more curious was a modern lady of leisure who confided sheepishly to her psychiatrist that she enjoyed many a relaxed afternoon rubbing the soles and toes of her feet with dog food and then inviting her two Pomeranians to lick it off. And not so long ago, a woman in her late thirties complained that her husband, a doctor, had amputated a number of her toes for 'sexual kicks'.

Foot sex seems firmly institutionalised and commercialised. In London, Berlin, Paris, Naples and Copenhagen, there are Palaces of Pedic Pleasure staffed by girls whose main qualification is that they shall possess beautiful, flexible feet and know how to use them in the associated erotic arts.

It becomes easier to understand why women have consciously – or unconsciously – gone to such lengths to beautify and to modify the feet, whatever the cost in pain, and to make them appear as dainty as possible.

It was in Medieval Europe, both as a declaration of fashionable elegance as well as of nobility that women had taken to appearing on tiptoe. Ladies of quality were wearing shoes so high in the sole that midgets were employed to walk either side of their unstable forms so that, from time to time, the ladies could rest their elbows on the little fellows' shoulders.

Walking tall was still popular in the sixteenth century when platform soles, or chopines, also served the more utilitarian purpose of raising women from contact with the slime and ordures of the street. They later became popular too for purely fashionable reasons, and wealthier women who would not dream of stepping abroad on filthy roads wore them as an attractive device to achieve an alluring wobble as they walked. Chopines might be anything from six to eighteen inches high, though thirty inches was not unusual. But they were a dangerous means of locomotion. Women fell from them. Pregnant women suffered miscarriages. Ben Jonson scoffed at them as 'treading on corked stilts at a prisoner's pace' whilst Shakespeare's Hamlet noted drily: 'Your ladyship is nearer to Heav'n than when I saw you last, by the height of your chopine.'

In Venice chopines were judged so very dangerous that as early as 1430 they were forbidden by law. But, naturally, women continued to wear them – occasionally summoning support to sustain a successful and conspicuous voyage across a drawing-room.

The truth was that men enjoyed watching the imperilled progress of ladies either in or

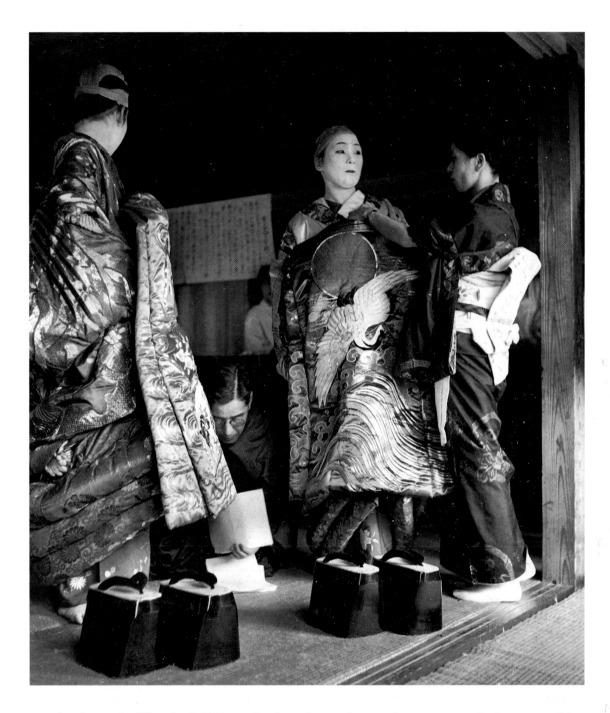

on chopines. As Havelock Ellis and others have observed, some men find a compelling attractiveness in lameness or uncertain gait in women. Perhaps this is why in Japan, there is an annual procession through the red-light district of Kyoto during which the great Whore of the Year is led through the streets, presumably exhausted, on twelve-inch-high chopines and supported on either side by two female apprentices.

A B O V E : Japanese geisha girls, highly esteemed professional entertainers, wearing foot-high lacquered chopines

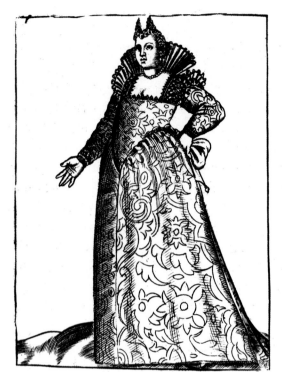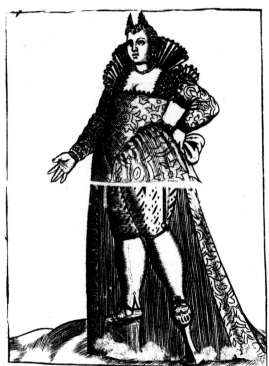

The truth revealed: how a Venetian courtesan managed to walk tall – she wore chopines

But though elevated walking – for whatever reason – had been popular for 3,000 years or more, it was only in the sixteenth century when Catherine de Médicis went to Paris to marry Henri II of France that high heels, as distinct from platform soles, first appeared. The petite Catherine took with her several pairs of shoes with heels designed specially for her by an inventive Italian. The idea was simply that she should appear taller and more elegant with the help of something more graceful and feminine than the solid chopine. The new high heels, delicate and slender, suited the purpose admirably, and the fact that they proved difficult to walk in only gave added lustre to their appeal. The restrictions they placed on movement simply helped to demonstrate that the wearer was pleasingly weak and helpless and more accustomed to leisure than to labour.

Soon they became *de rigueur* for the aristocracy and the expression 'well-heeled' was born. Women liked them, well aware of the flirtatious appeal their unstable tottering offered. Men liked them too, fascinated by the way they caused the female hips to sway, pushed out the posterior, and gave the bust a provocative forward thrust.

Indeed, for the watching male, the pleasure was doubled – not only was he captivated by the seductive swaying across the room of a lady on slender spikes but he also had the excitement of being constantly on the *qui-vive* for the possibility of a quick protective conquest should she stumble. The chance of rescuing a 'fallen' woman was an enticing prospect for both parties. It was really quite intriguing that in one small progress across a crowded room a woman might become both predator and prey.

But though the new high heels had, without a doubt, come to stay, there were many who disapproved. Mr Punch was still protesting about tight shoes and high heels in the 1870s: 'So let them [feet and toes] be deformed and crumpled up by these instruments of torture and grow misshapen and distorted like the feet of the Chinese. Deformity becomes a proof of fashionable breeding and it is better to be hideous than not to dress à la mode.'

But neither the caustic observations of *Punch* nor warnings from the medical profession, nor all the cautionary tales from all corners of the world have ever influenced the fashionable woman's choice of footwear. In 1987, Dolcis sold 260,000 pairs of stilettos.

'They're dangerous . . . but white stilettos will be the most bought-out shoe style in the British high street this summer,' predicted one fashion magazine in June 1988. Dr Alan M. Davis of the Health Education Council added his warning: 'Wearing stiletto heels can cause damage to your feet, legs and posture. Sloping toes crushed into pointed spaces will develop calluses, bunions and corns or even the dreaded hammer-toe syndrome.'

He will be totally ignored. The majority of women still accept that their 'best' shoes will not be comfortable, that for a wedding or any great occasion women must look 'right' above all else and then expect to grit their teeth and bear the consequences. Almost always high heels are part of that 'rightness'. They remain the hall-mark of the elegant woman. They flatter the leg; they have sex appeal; men like them. As a famous madame of a New Orleans brothel once said in the 1850s: 'We found we could double the fees when the girls sashayed around in those high heels. It gave a look of class to the ass. The men went crazy just watching. . . . They drank more, stayed longer and came back more often.'

10. THE PSYCHOLOGY OF BEAUTY

Some lovers of beauty, like the Greeks of classical times, declared our sense of beauty to be instinctive, something we recognise quite clearly when we see it. They believed, like Sir Joshua Reynolds, that things of beauty have a clearly definable nature – that they obey fixed mathematical rules of shape and proportion. Hogarth, on the other hand, was not impressed by these classical rules, but believed instead that beauty's essential constituent was nothing more than the serpentine line – his famous 'wavy line of beauty' – sometimes seen in the outline of a particularly beautiful face or figure. Others have stressed the importance of perfect symmetry or balance – an idea rejected by Sir Francis Bacon who emphasised instead the peculiar fascination of slight imperfection. 'There is no perfect beauty', he said, 'that hath not some strangeness in the proportion'.

But this preoccupation with the fixed characteristics or 'formula' for beauty surely misses the point; beauty takes so many forms which can differ in so many ways. Much depends, for example, on where in the world you happen to be; ideas of beauty are so remarkably diverse in different cultures. Evidence from the other side of the world can leave us in no doubt that ideals of beauty differ radically from one country to another. This can only mean that our standards of beauty must, to a large degree, be 'trained' into us by the society we live in, by family and by those closest to us. André Gide went further; he said that we are trained not only by the people – but also by the things – we see around us. Even the art we look at changes our standards. 'Sunsets', he said, 'have never been the same since Turner.'

It follows, therefore, that for those of us who are of a mind to 'improve' ourselves, an important part of becoming beautiful – of becoming attractive – would consist in enhancing and developing those special aspects of ourselves which our own particular society happens to admire, has been trained to admire. And this applies not only to physical things like face and figure, thinness or fatness, but to psychological characteristics – such as temperament and character, attitudes and indeed many of our everyday habits and styles of behaviour. And of course the things which our own society trains us to admire are quite likely to change a good deal from age to age, and even, under the powerful pressures of fashion, from year to year. Hogarth's 'curvaceous' principle was temporarily forgotten in the 1920s.

And there are individual preferences to consider; if we explore people's minds carefully enough we discover that ideals of beauty differ a great deal not only from place to place, and age to age, but also from person to person.

It was the Scottish philosopher David Hume who probably came nearest to the truth

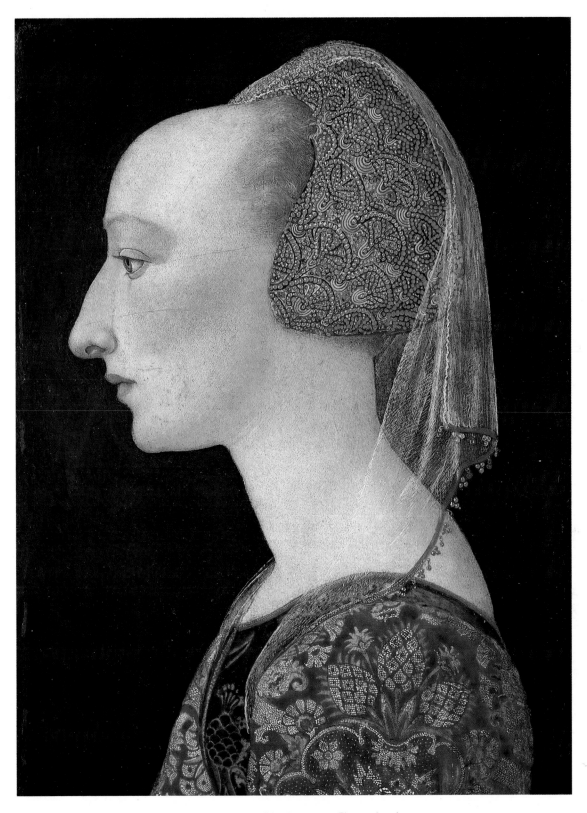

A fifteenth-century ideal: young Florentine beauty

about this when he first talked about 'the eye of the beholder'. It is in our minds, he explained, that beauty is created. 'Beauty is not a quality in things themselves, it exists merely in the mind that contemplates them, and each mind perceives a different beauty.'

According to this view, people, and their faces, and their bodies, are in many respects like the inkblots of the psychologist's test – hardly more than triggers which set off the creations of our personal imaginations. The faces of the people we meet are, on this view, nothing more than a set of hooks on which we can hang our personal sentiments and prejudices. The idea is simply that we 'create' the person that we want to see and need to see. This is why there is such extraordinary variation in different people's perceptions and descriptions of the same individual. Which, of course, is just as well: at least everybody has a chance of being attractive to somebody!

Many famous beauties of the past have been described as 'fascinating', 'mysterious', 'elusive'. This reminds us that one important element in the complex experience of beauty is a certain indefiniteness or a lack of clarity in the image that we perceive, and most importantly, perhaps, a certain enigmatic quality. Leonardo's 'Mona Lisa' supports an infinity of possibilities. Impressionist painters grasped this principle; their beauties were often vague, ill-defined, unclear in outline. We each interpret them in our own special way. We make of them what we will. We are able, in fantasy at least, to convert them into anything our heart happens – at this particular moment – to desire. Skilled photographers have long known how to fabricate this powerful effect with soft focus lenses, leaving maximum scope for ample 'conversion' by the eye and the mind of the beholder. Cecil Beaton's special genius was to achieve the same mental effect by clever choice of environmental setting and background and dress. At deeper, less conscious levels too this same principle holds. There is a deep fascination in ambiguity; the human puzzle rivets our attention. Modern pop-stars exploit the fascinations of ambiguity by deliberately making themselves 'hard to place'. Boy George, for a moment at least, keeps us guessing, notably about gender. Designers of fashion too, perhaps without realising it, are often conspicuously successful when they oscillate our minds in this way, juxtaposing female and male stimuli, adding a great deal to their creations' appeal. Even broad shoulders on female dress enjoyed a certain, though predictably short, vogue for this reason. On the stage, female impersonators have long traded on this effect. And among the immortals Garbo seemed even more compellingly beautiful playing both sexes in 'Queen Christina'. But Greta Garbo, according to Kenneth Clark, 'arguably one of the most beautiful women who has ever lived,' possessed a face which just happened to possess in the highest degree this magical quality of 'convertibility'. Bergman and Dietrich too had this wonderful gift. The viewer's hungry imagination could transform their faces into almost anything the heart desired.

Our experience of beauty can have some curious – and quite unexpected – origins;

OPPOSITE : Greta Garbo: 'arguably one of the most beautiful women who have ever lived'

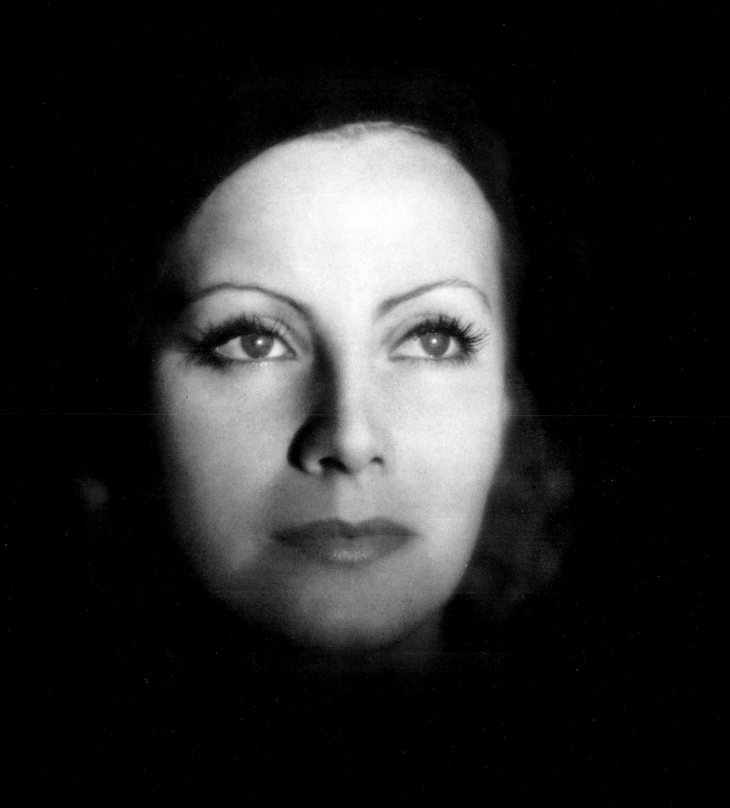

nostalgia, for example, can play a very important role. Our early memories of parents and loved ones can sometimes influence our mature adult preferences. Happy and rewarding experiences in the bosom of the family can predispose us, by the powerful mechanism of conditioning, to prefer people who remind us, by some aspect of their physical appearance, of our own family. And since we ourselves inevitably possess at least some of our family characteristics then it must follow that we are instinctively attracted to people who are physically, in some respects, like ourselves. This seemingly narcissistic preference for carbon copies of ourselves even extends to psychological characteristics; we prefer people who share our attitudes, values, and prejudices – and especially our personality traits. We can understand such people better. There are no awkward surprises; we can predict their behaviour better. They are more comfortable to be with. We can easily get to like them – and to regard them as good and wholesome. Ambrose Bierce's joking definition of 'admiration' as 'our polite recognition of another's similarity to ourselves' has more than a little truth in real life.

One American sociologist, Frumkin, believed that our experience of beauty was intimately related to our sexual urges – that the feeling of 'beauty' is generated when we recognise in people what he called their 'sexual aptitude' – their adequacy for their natural erotic and reproductive role. Freud expressed a similar notion. Havelock Ellis had much the same idea when he suggested that, for many people, a pregnant woman was movingly beautiful for this very reason. It was Charles Darwin, of course, who emphasised the crucial importance of the more 'obvious' and visible physical differences between the sexes in bringing about, in both human and animal kingdoms, that most important function of all – reproduction – without which life could not go on. If this is true then it follows that, in the presence of that instinct to reproduce, simple sex differences of whatever kind will become in themselves highly attractive; and there can be no doubt that an important fraction of the image and experience of beauty is often created by the perception of these biological differences in the opposite sex. It follows that the female's naturally-smaller stature, more rounded, less muscular frame, less muscular, less mobile face, smaller nose, and smoother skin will always excite many male admirers. And it follows too that any artificial device or embellishment, whether clothing or jewellery or cosmetic substance which exaggerates, or which merely creates the illusion of, these natural differences will necessarily increase overall attractiveness to the opposite sex. There is much to be exploited here – the contrast effects, for example, of the large hat or coiffure flatteringly miniaturising the face – or of flowing mobile hair, reducing, again by visual contrast, the apparent movements of the facial musculature. The apparent movement, relative to one another, of veil and face may again impart a feminising placidity to the face for the same reason.

Yet though the large muscular male with hairy face and deep voice may have been designed by nature to stir female hearts, this can only be the beginning of the story of sexual attractiveness. Psychological qualities too are important, as recent reliable research has shown; a good deal of the female's excitement evidently comes not so much from viewing male physique as from awareness and satisfaction in beholding his character and personality – strength of will rather than strength of arm. Indeed, it is now clear that many females actively dislike exaggeratedly-muscular body-builders. It looks, therefore, as though the male who is set on improving his sex appeal has a problem on his hands – his chief task is not so much to enhance the physical as to create convincing images of the psychological – of the true, sterling, reliable and interesting character beneath the outward display which may, initially of course, have attracted her attention. Illusions, too, of such desirable personality qualities can, of course, be created by skilful choice of dress and 'personal décor'.

The enigma of sex appeal takes yet another twist when we discover that the male view of female attractiveness may not be the same as the female view. Men and women frequently have quite different emphases in their conceptions of 'masculinity' and 'femininity'. The writers' recent research, for example, has shown that many women attach much more importance to their own smooth and clear complexions than do men. Males, on the other hand, are more preoccupied with females' delicate features and with their hair. On the question of masculinity too, this particular research showed interesting disagreements: females looked for firm jaw, strong mouth, facial hair and stubbly chin while males were more concerned with their own hair length and style – a matter of surprisingly little concern to the females. There was complete unanimity among both males and females however about the importance of youth, and its close neighbour health, in producing an impression of attractiveness. And those frequent attributes of youth, delicate features and clear eyes, were often mentioned, as indeed were the psychological, and not just the physical, qualities associated with youth – innocence, directness and lack of guile. And, perhaps surprisingly, men were much less attracted by slimness than women seem to think they are. But perhaps this is not so surprising, since, after all, as Darwin would have explained, a major biological difference in women is their softness and roundness, qualities hardly to be found in the successful slimming fanatic.

Perhaps we get closer to the heart of the mystery of sexual attraction when we listen to sex researchers like the American husband and wife team Masters and Johnson who have found by careful and sensitive interviewing that men and women are quite different in their dependence on visual sexual images. It is mainly men and not women who are sexually aroused by what they see. For men, the visual image, whether in reality or fantasy, seems paramount in sexual arousal. For women sexual sights are much less exciting, though male strip shows are sometimes said to be mildly diverting.

One must assume therefore that it is women, rather than men, who need to have a special care for their visual appearance if they wish to give a helping hand to Nature, or even if they simply want to reap the humbler but highly gratifying rewards of being attractive.

But it is nonsense to suggest that our pursuit of elegance and beauty is only, or even mainly, sexually driven. Sexual fulfilment is only one of the factors in personal happiness. We are, after all, social animals. Adler said we spend our lives pursuing our one major preoccupation – finding ways to relate to and make contact with people, to influence them, to impress them, to make ourselves attractive to them (and not necessarily in any sexual sense). We are certainly prepared, he said, to go to a great deal of effort, and if needs be, a good deal of suffering, to achieve these objectives. We must, above all, chase away our inferiority feelings by proving to ourselves that we count for something and that we are capable of attracting attention. Tolstoy put it another way: 'Nothing', he said, 'has so marked an influence on the direction of a man's mind as his appearance, and not his appearance itself, so much as his conviction that it is attractive or unattractive.'

Many modern psychologists would go further; our whole happiness, they say, depends crucially on our ability to maintain a positive self-image. And since a significant part of our self image is inevitably centred on our appearance it is natural enough that we should be concerned, perhaps even preoccupied, with our attractiveness and the possibilities of its enhancement.

11. THE REASONS WHY

A WOMAN'S VIEW

The writer Alexander Black commenting in 1923 on the vanity of women – and in most part complaining about their slavish devotion to fashion and their painstaking use of cosmetics – was forced to confess that both men and women make extraordinary sacrifices in the interests of their appearance. 'A man doesn't feel dressed until he is throttled by a collar. A woman doesn't feel fashionable unless something hurts. It is at the excess point that fashion-consciousness begins,' he said.

In the past extravagant attempts to achieve beauty by dangerous experimentation, or by following the excesses of fashion have applied more to the rich than to the poor; the poor have rarely had the time to experiment with cosmetics, nor the resources to keep up with fashion's exclusivity. Exclusiveness is indissolubly linked to costliness. When garments become cheaper to make they lose – by some perverse miracle – their fashionable charms. Witness what happened to the crinoline. The invention of the sewing-machine in the late 1850s quickly brought this labour-intensive garment within the reach of all. More and more women were able to make skirts as outrageously voluminous as those of the wealthy. Once this became possible, the crinoline fell out of fashion. Cosmetics have experienced a similar fate. When lipsticks became available at Woolworth's in the 1920s, there was an immediate call for an expensive range of more subtle colours to distinguish mill-girls from miladies.

Nowadays, haute-couture is rapidly translated into street fashion. Any woman, however modest her means, can aspire to being fashionable. It is true there persists the ridiculous, universal requirement of a wand-slim body on which to drape the season's style, but shapes and fabrics are not so rigidly prescribed as they used to be. There is so much more scope for women, however modest their means, to cut a dash.

But why have so many generations of women been so prepared to be such slaves to fashion, whatever the cost in discomfort? Is there some magical force in novelty which has motivated them – or has fashion simply been the catalyst, releasing and interpreting some deeper feminine need?

There can be no general answer. One woman's motives for beauty-seeking are not another's: different personalities are subject to different impulses. Different nationalities, too, will have their own special priorities and values. And the changing social pressures of different centuries necessarily affect women's behaviour. The women of polite society in the eighteenth and nineteenth centuries must undoubtedly have felt a greater pressure to conformity than their counterparts today.

There have been great variations too in women's scope and freedom to indulge their whims. But fairly consistently, women have been told that it is a woman's mission in life to be beautiful. Social traditions have generally supported this objective and consequently there has always been a tendency to accept a greater degree of narcissism in women than in men.

Again, almost all women have an instinctive love of variety and desire for change. But even if we accept this as a fact of life, the question remains – why have they chosen their own bodies as the medium for satisfying these needs? Psychologist Seymour Fisher believes he has the answer; women have to maintain a flexible attitude towards the body, he says, because their biological natures force so many obligatory rituals on them – menstruation, for example, and their unique potential for becoming pregnant. Unable to beat these inexorable rhythms, they act out in public, through clothes and make-up, their 'private sense of being in bodily flux'. And they do this with considerable enthusiasm. Indeed, says Fisher, 'They approach their body topography with some of the same zest for novelty as is shown by the explorer looking for new territory.'

The psychologist Karl Menninger, on the other hand, talks of 'focal suicide'. He insists that all women suffer from it – this burning desire to alter parts of the body. And they do this, he says, in order to add erotic dimensions to their charms.

Certainly, most women, offered the chance of an exciting change which promises to make them more attractive, will yield to the temptation to experiment. There will always be the risk of failure, or even the possibility of ridicule. But there will also be the excitement of uncertainty and the thrill of danger. Experimentation itself has such a stimulating effect on the senses, an excitement all its own.

And there is always the lure of hope – hope for better things, hope for greater beauty perhaps. It is not always easy – and a good deal of patience may be necessary – but it was Helena Rubinstein's belief that whatever the foundation, beauty can always be gained by carefully-chosen cosmetics, and a certain amount of persistence. 'There are no ugly women,' she said, 'only lazy ones.' With such a seductive call to arms, what woman would not be prepared to jump to it and apply herself energetically to the business of self-improvement? If defeating ugliness simply means conquering laziness (and purchasing Rubinstein products) then surely this is not too high a price to pay?

But more than honest effort and persistence is required if ugly ducklings are to be made into real swans and not just nicer-looking ducklings. Most women, after all, want to be swans. So their efforts have amounted to much more than just avoiding laziness. As we have seen, they frequently amounted to self-torture. Some writers on the psychology of beauty have gone so far as to label it 'masochism'. So here we have a new twist – the suggestion that women's relentless pursuit of beautification is, in fact, the indulgence of the peculiarly exquisite enjoyment of self-punishment. The idea is that women actually enjoy pain.

Freud believed that we have a strong death wish which prompts us to assault our bodies, but not all modern psychologists share this view.

A number of women have confessed to pleasure in suffering. The American rock singer, Debbie Harry, talking about the tiresome hairs on her legs, explained how it felt as she removed them: 'I pluck them out one at a time,' she said. 'I enjoy the pain.' Journalist and pundit Malcolm Muggeridge found himself marvelling at American women: 'How they mortify the flesh in order to make it appetizing. Their beauty is a vast industry, their enduring allure a discipline which nuns and athletes might find excessive.'

Contemporary actresses and models have been heard to comment that it is also a question of public relations, because 'an aura of martyrdom is good publicity'.

The much more prosaic urge to keep age at bay seems a likelier reason. Because the trouble with age is . . . it shows. As one wise sixteenth-century philosopher suggested: 'A beautiful woman should break her mirror early' – advice which his Queen, Elizabeth I, took very much to heart, banishing all the mirrors from her household. Why should it have mattered so much? Were the ravages of age too terrible even for the strongest woman of her century?

But then, the problem is not just an aesthetic one. Our face is our greatest ambassador: nakedly it confronts the world. Regrettably, as we know, it is all too revealing. In women it often reflects, unkindly, deep biological changes – the menopausal retreat of certain feminine hormones, stark signals of a declining sexual attractiveness. Like a broadsheet written in upper case, the elderly female face reveals to the world that here is a woman fecundity has pensioned off. The ageing face proclaims diminished power – diminished power to function as a woman, to participate, to make a real impact, to 'have a voice', to command respect. It is easy enough to see why business executives strain to look young and fit and why they are prepared to spend such large sums on cosmetic surgery. It is even easier to see why ageing film stars submit to skin-grafting and face-lifts to retain their image of youthful sex and vigour.

Perhaps we could deal better with the problem of ageing, however, if age were simply our own affair. But in many ways it is not. We interact with others. And other people respond to us – initially at least – according to what we look like. As moralists tell us, it may be character that really matters. But we have to get through the appearance barrier before we can appreciate the person beneath. This difficulty was made very clear by Doreen Trust, who opened what she described as the world's first Guidance Centre for the Disfigured in 1983. As she pointed out, the message from an ugly person's face so often seems to be an unpleasant one. So we turn away. We all seem to have fallen for that old cliché about beauty being good, and ugliness evil.

Not surprising then that with so much at stake women have always paid particular attention to their appearance. Indeed, a woman's 'value', quite unfairly, has often seemed to depend almost entirely on her superficial looks. If she attracted attention, it was usually through her beauty. How many millions of plain women must have fretted in the knowledge that something quite spectacular would need to happen if they were going to get themselves noticed at all?

Sometimes, though, the need to be noticed springs simply from the desire to communicate a message – perhaps about class, status, wealth, competence or intelligence, or just from a desire for triumphant declaration that we are in total command and total control of our environment.

Elizabeth I was prepared to stagger under a great load of ceremonial dress; she left no-one in doubt about her rank. Even today, in the workplace, a catering manageress will wear a stiffly formal dress and crippling high-heeled shoes to express her authority as she moves about among her waitresses, more comfortably attired and certainly more comfortably shod. To hold down the job a woman may feel she needs to appear younger, more alert, more energetic. Uncomfortable 'status' garments, a punishing diet – even cosmetic surgery – begin to seem very worth while. Declarations about wealth and class are often attempted through jewellery and ostentatiously expensive clothes. Unfortunately, diamonds and designer-labels tend to sit uncomfortably and unnaturally on over-ambitious wearers. The outcome, all too often, is the uneasy, haggard face of striving – the very opposite of effortless elegance.

And yet we all need to express ourselves. To do so is healthy and natural. The problem is, what are we trying to express? The real person that we truly are? Or some fantasy figure that we would so much like to be? Or even the figure we think we ought to be?

For all women there exists a half-hidden image of what she could look like, if only she tried – the special day when, fleetingly seen through a kindly mirror, she caught herself looking almost attractive . . . the memorable wedding-day photograph to which a generous soft lens gave miraculous beauty. The conviction that she could be beautiful, if only she made sufficient effort – perhaps by greater dedication, a new diet or new regime. However punishing, all this effort seems so worth while.

For many, though, there is a greater tyrant – the drive to achieve aesthetic perfection. Inspiration may come from the glamorous stars of television or film, or from art and literature. These images can powerfully shape our style, our clothes, our make-up or even our mannerisms. At the same time, they may work against our real strengths and be quite out of character with our true personality.

In much the same way, the woman who attempts to live up to the highly specific notions of beauty held by the man in her life may well find herself in trouble. In trying to match up to the ideal woman of his fantasies she may be stretching nature far beyond its reasonable limits. Throughout history, 'He' has been cast as the hunter and warrior. 'She', on the other hand, has played the part of the home-maker and child-bearer. Her fecund shape, seen so often in primitive sculpture and cave-painting, shows the persistent, universal stereotype of earth-mother figure with large buttocks, breasts and belly. Undoubtedly, this image looms large in the male unconscious, as C. G. Jung has made clear; this is the form and function which woman needs in order to fulfil her female destiny. But much more than this is demanded. In addition to these serviceable utilitarian characteristics, many men have also required of their women the qualities of gentle submissiveness, loyal supportiveness and, of course, perfect beauty, examples of which are threateningly all around. Women have always been eager to fulfil these needs as best they can. They have always taken pleasure in attracting attention and in captivating male admirers. Generation after generation have diligently sought that small but important element of this – the secret of 'sex appeal'.

But not all men continue to like the same things. Historical record shows that males have been influenced by widely-varying, and sometimes highly ephemeral ideals of perfection. There have been great swings in tastes over the centuries. Sometimes – as we can see from fourteenth-century paintings – the desire has been for near-bosomless, pregnant-looking ladies, sometimes again for the riper-looking ladies admired by Rubens, and then, again quite differently, for the boneless, boyish beauties of the nineteen-twenties.

There have been continuous shifts too, in the female focus of male attention; woman's sex-appeal has centred sometimes in her flowing hair, and sometimes in her dazzlingly pale complexion and sparkling eyes, and sometimes again in her tiny waist, or her dainty feet, or her hips, or her bosom, or yet at other times, even her lack of bosom: what the psychologist, J. C. Flugel, has referred to as the 'shifting erogenous zones'.

One thing only has remained constant: whatever the requirement – banishing or building up the bosom, painfully squeezing the waist, compressing the feet – women have always met the need with determination and very little questioning; underpinning all beautifying effort has been the stoic philosophy that one must suffer to be beautiful – 'Il faut souffrir pour être belle'.

A MAN'S VIEW

It is strange to discover just how similar are the motivations of men and women in pursuing beauty and elegance. Still the same vanity, still the same desire to attract . . . still the same urge to attain an ideal image firmly fixed in the mind.

There are differences, of course, in male psychology. For many men, pride in strength and physique is prominent. The need for influence, prestige and power is so much more deeply rooted. Every badge of rank – every proof of power, success and achievement – is eagerly sought and by no means, as is so often suggested, just to appeal to the opposite sex.

For the well-to-do, exclusive fashion has always provided ample opportunity for aggressive ostentation and display of riches and success even if (as so often with women too) it has entailed uncomfortable and time-consuming rituals in dressing-rooms. Stuffed shirts, starched collars, body-belts, and cummerbunds are not the easiest of dinner companions yet they continue to be tolerated.

The pursuit of youth can take a harsh toll, especially for those men who are sensitive to the ageing implications of their white or balding heads. Again, the determination that many men show to lose weight requires no less dedication and sacrifice than women's. The current vogue for the slim 'New Man' has given rise to disastrously increasing numbers suffering from anorexia – no longer medically regarded, as it once was, as an exclusively female problem. And joggers and muscle-men tend to push their bodies to medically dangerous extremes. A new fascination with the ambiguities of androgyny – so well illustrated by Boy George – and with interestingly-shocking images borrowed from the world of 'Pop' – has provided a new set of problems both in dress and in male cosmetic treatments – not least the courage to wear them.

Cosmetic surgery, on the other hand, can often be passed off by men as professional necessity. But does holding down the job really require the face to be lifted, the jowls to be cropped? Or is this a convenient rationalisation for old-fashioned vanity?

Underlying many men's efforts is perhaps that deepest of all male preoccupations – the idea of youthful virility. Images of male attractiveness, virility and masculinity are for the male closely intertwined – much more so than the corresponding qualities in women. Youth, vigour, strength, the dark stubble-growth, free from any trace of grey, the hairy face and chest, are well-worn clichés of masculinity but many men will go to considerable trouble to display them. And there are those who will gladly submit themselves to glandular intervention – even surgery – to keep the flag of youth flying. Though men's conception of male attractiveness is not the same as women's (as we saw in Chapter 10) most men have a clear enough image of masculinity in their mind – and many are prepared to go to great lengths to project that particular personal image however unusual it may be.

12. SLAVES TO FASHION:
A CONCLUSION

'It is a perfectly natural desire to admire and often to exaggerate whatever nature may have given us,' Charles Darwin wrote. It would certainly not be natural if we should ever cease to be interested in making ourselves more beautiful.

Looking our best is satisfying, making the most of ourselves, exhilarating. The trouble is, we are often tempted to do a good deal more than this, seeking transformations which go far beyond the enhancement of our natural assets. Sometimes we attempt radical change. We reach for the impossible. To change from black skin to white, from a 28-inch to a 16-inch waist, from a normal foot to a 3-inch travesty is flying in the face of Nature. Inevitably there are problems. And the bigger the gap between what is aspired to and what is attainable, the greater the problems will be. The wider the gulf between aspiration and practical reality, the more intense the suffering.

The temptations, though, are often very hard to resist. We live in the chaos of a communications explosion. Commercial messages are hurled at us from all sides. Advertisers tell us what we want to hear – that we can transform our whole appearance if only we will buy this or that product, follow this or that cult, theory or regime. Repetition after repetition eventually convinces us that beauty is what the media say it is – and achieving it is simple, straightforward. Yet there is an almost monotonous sameness about the models they employ. We are bombarded with stereotypes. And the trouble with these stereotypes is that whilst they may vary superficially they are always underpinned by two seemingly mandatory fundamentals: that our faces must be beautiful and our bodies must not be fat.

Every day we are relentlessly exposed to examples of beauty we are told we should aspire to. And these ideal faces paraded before us become more and more unrealistically 'perfect', the ideal bodies are excruciatingly thin. ('You can never be too rich or too thin,' said the Duchess of Windsor.) Even when fashion does decide to acknowledge the curves and contours of the female body it goes to extremes in promoting enormous bosoms, the tiniest of waists, and long, long legs.

For all of us, the scope for alteration is now considerable. With sophisticated technology we have almost reached the stage where, given the licence to do so and the necessary ethical abandon, we could produce a gene-guaranteed, sex-arranged human being of unmatched perfection, nurturing and trimming it to a pre-determined ideal by any necessary cosmetic surgery. And then, no doubt, maintain its eternal youth by regular injections of animal cells at some hi-tech Swiss clinic.

When Mrs Patrick Campbell had the bright idea of proposing marriage to George Bernard Shaw with the suggestion that their progeny would have his brain and her beauty, he countered with: 'Reflect for a moment Madam, on the fate of that unfortunate infant should by mischance he be born with your brains and my looks.'

We are almost capable now of overcoming such a 'mischance'. But even that might not satisfy us. In our visually obsessed society we aim even higher. We demand both brains and beauty, at least from those at the top. It is not enough to be good at a job, we also have to present the right image; politicians nowadays are judged as much by their television appearance as by their policies. And down the pecking order, there are still so many rewards for attractiveness. Juries will acquit us more often, or give us lighter sentences, if we happen to be good-looking. People in general will like us better – they assign better personalities to those of us who are attractive. Even getting a job may depend on it. In 1982 alone, 1,000 Japanese students submitted themselves to cosmetic surgery to improve their chances of employment – and these figures are from one hospital alone. In 1988, a directive to managers of a Japanese factory in Wales required them to hire 'presentable female staff who are not fat'.

Yet recognition – even a celebration – of individuality has characterised social life in the 1980s. Roles have been reversed, priorities altered. The sexes have adventured ever more freely into each other's territories. Some women are flourishing in executive areas hitherto exclusively male. Some men find themselves genuinely more at home and relaxed in domestic situations. And plenty of women – fulfilling themselves in ways they never before dreamed possible – are making it clear that they have better things to do with their time than sit in front of mirrors and count calories. Whilst interested in enhancing attractiveness, they are no longer prepared to put up with so much discomfort in pursuit of it.

Female 'liberation', for all its false starts, has brought to women the privilege of at last being 'themselves'. And the spin-off for men is that they too are able to be so much more 'themselves'. Those men who prefer colourful dress, who wish to grow long hair, have it permanently waved, wear earrings, are no longer looked at askance.

The new egalitarian spirit has brought about a refreshing mix of male and female ideals and targets in this whole complicated area of attractiveness. Just one manifestation of this is the growing fascination with androgyny. Androgyny is, at the very least, a welcome break-away from stereotypy. The Punks, however outrageous they sometimes seemed, were attempting vigorously to express themselves.

It is tempting to speculate that the social upheavals of the past three decades may well bring about even more profound changes in attitudes to beauty and physical appearance in the coming twenty-first century.

Will there be one of those sudden shifts so common throughout history, when the majority of women – whatever their personal motivation – will return once more to the old, demanding standards of stereotyped femininity? Or will more and more women hold fast to the idea of beauty without effort, and self-expression as the keynote of their philosophy?

And there is now one further, quite new factor to consider; the sex-balance of the population is changing. In the past, there have always been more boys born than girls but more of them have died in infancy. Improved medical care is now keeping more of these young boys alive – with the result that in the 1970s, the young male population began to overtake that of young females. Already in the 1980s, according to United Nations figures, there are 30 million more young males than young females in the world (all aged 23 years and below) and the gap is widening each year. In Europe alone, there are 2 million more young men than women: in the U.S.A. 3 million. So the traditional shortfall of young adult males has been transformed into a shortfall of young adult females – which leads to the intriguing speculation: how far will tomorrow's men go in advancing their attempts to express themselves more liberally, more colourfully, and necessarily with more effort? Could it be men's turn next to carry on the tradition of more than two thousand years of the tyranny of beauty?

SOURCES

1. STARVING FOR STYLE

Eichenbaum, Luise & Orbach, Susie, *Understanding Women*, 1983.
Edwards, Ann, *Judy Garland*, 1975.
Gatty, Charles Neilson, *The Elephant That Swallowed a Nightingale*, 1981.
Jaeger, Gustav (trnsl. Tomalin, Lewis, R. S.), *Health Culture*, 1907.
Stancioff, Nadia, *Maria Callas Remembered*, 1988.
Conley, Rosemary, *Hip and Thigh Diet*, 1988.
Katahn, Martin, *The Rotation Diet*, 1988.
Eyton, Audrey, *The F-Plan Diet*, 1982.
Eyton, Audrey, *The Easier F-Plan Diet* (combined edition), 1987.
Diamond, Harvey & Marilyn, *Fit for Life*, 1985 (paperback 1987).
Black, Gayle, *The Sun Sign Diet*, 1986.
Howard, Alan, *The Cambridge Diet*, 1985.
French, Barbara, *Coping With Bulimia*, 1987.
Roche, Louise, *Glutton For Punishment*, 1984.
Orbach, Susie, *Fat is a Feminist Issue*, 1978.
Roberts, Nancy, *Breaking All the Rules, Feeling Good and Looking Great No Matter What your Size*,
    1985.
Gillie, Oliver, News item *The Sunday Times*, 7.10.84.
Beller, Anne Scott, *Fat and Thin*, 1977.
MacLeod, Sheila, *The Art of Starvation*, 1981.
Summers, A., *Goddess (The Secret Lives of Marilyn Monroe)*, 1985.

2. THE BEWILDERING BOSOM

Beaton, C., *The Glass of Fashion*, 1953.
Plat, Sir Hugh, *Delightes for Ladies*, 1627.
Pignatelli, Luciana, *The Beautiful People's Beauty Book*, 1971.
Greer, Germaine, *The Female Eunuch*, 1971.
Caseby, Jo., news item, *Western Mail*, 7.12.88.

3. DRESSED TO KILL

Waugh, Norah, *Corsets and Crinolines*, 1954.
Rudofsky, B., *The Fashionable Body*, 1971.
Poiret, Paul, *My First 50 Years*, 1907.
Laver, James, *Concise History of Costume*, 1969.
Limner, Luke (John Leighton), *Madre Natura Versus the Moloch of Fashion*, 1874.
Kunzle, David, *Fashion and Fetishism*, 1982.

Canter Cremers-van der Does, Eline, *The Agony of Fashion*, 1980.
Wroblewski, Chris, *Tattoo*, 1987.
Burchett, George, *Memoirs of a Tattooist*, 1958.
Bell, Joy Ann & Carter, George, 'Tight Girdle or Sömmering's Syndrome', *New England Jnl Medicine*, 1973.
Flugel, J. C., *The Psychology of Clothes*, 1950.

4. THE FACE: CHANGING THE COLOUR

Coleman, Vernon with Coleman Margaret, *Face Values*, 1981.
Jackson, Michael, *Moonwalk*, 1988.
Brown, Peter Harry & Brown, Pamela Ann, *The MGM Girls*, 1984.
Higham, Charles & Moseley, Roy, *Merle*, 1983.
Colby, A., *Anita Colby's Beauty Book*, 1958.
Harry, R. G., *Cosmetic Materials*, 1963.
Staffe, Baroness, *The Lady's Dressing Room*, 1892.
Wilkinson, D. S., 'The History and Hazards of Cosmetics', (In Michaelmas *Murmer*) 1967.
Hoey, Mrs Cashel, *Ten Centuries of Toilette* (trnsl. from French by Robida, A.), 1892.
Corson, Richard, *Fashions in Makeup*, 1972.
Williams, Neville, *Powder and Paint*, 1957.
Boy George, *Fashion and Makeup Book*, 1984.
Collingbourne, Huw, *Madonna*, 1987.
Maxwell Hudson, Clare, *Kaleidoscope of Beauty*, 1968.
Polhemus, Ted & Procter, Lynn, *Pop Styles*, 1984.
Le Camus, Antoine, *The Art of Preserving Beauty*, 1754.
Griffin, John, *Black Like Me*, 1960.
Halsell, Grace, *Soul Sister*, 1970.
Angeloglou, M., *A History of Makeup*, 1970.
Kenton, Leslie, *The Joy of Beauty*, 1983.
'Bandung File', Channel 4 TV, 21.6.88.
Beresford, D., *Guardian* article, 15.5.87.
H.M. Stationery Office, *Consumer Protection* (The Cosmetic Products Safety Regulations), 1984.
The London Magazine, article, 1768.
The Lady's Magazine, articles 1776 & Feb. 1793.

5. THE FACE: CHANGING THE TEXTURE

Joyce, T. Athol and Thomas, N. W. (Ed.), *Women of All Nations*, 1909.
Sylvia, *Sylvia's Book of the Toilet*, 1881.
Jeamson, J., *Artificiall Embellishments of Arts Best Directions*, 1665.
Gerard, John, *Gerard's Herbal*, 1597.
Sheba, *Women Who Fascinate and Why*, 1924.
Marks, Prof. Ronald, *The Sun and Your Skin*, 1988.

Fitzsimons, Carmel, *The Observer* (news item), 22.6.86.
Montagu, Lady Mary Wortley, *Letters*, December 1716.
Best, magazine, April 1988.
Levine, Robert, *Joan Collins Superstar*, 1985.
Brain, Robert, *The Decorated Body*, 1979.
Morris, Desmond, *Bodywatching*, 1985.

6. THE FACE: PERSUASIVE PARTS

Chapkis, Wendy, *Beauty Secrets*, 1988.
Woodforde, J., *The Strange Story of False Teeth*, 1968.
Loren, Sophia, *Women and Beauty*, 1984.
Rhodes, Russell R., *Man at his Best*, 1975.
Bulwer, J., *Anthropometamorphosis*, 1650.
Lavater, J. C., *Essays in Physiognomy*, 1789.
Tommaseo, *Moral Thoughts (Studi Morali)*, 1858.

7. THE FACE: CHANGING THE SHAPE

Felstein, Ivor, *A Change of Face and Figure*, 1971.
Gardiner, Leslie E., *Faces Figures and Feelings*, 1959.
Rees, Thos. D., *Cosmetic Facial Surgery*, 1973.

8. CROWNS OF GLORY: THE HAIR

Corson, R., *Fashions in Hair*, 1965.
Cooper, Wendy, *Hair*, 1971.
Sagay, Esi, *African Hairstyles*, 1983–87.
Sassoon, Vidal, *Sorry I Kept You Waiting Madam*, 1968.
Knight, Nick, *Skinhead*, 1982.
Charlesworth, Chris, *Elton John*, 1986.
Currie, David, *David Bowie*, 1985.
Woodforde, J., *The Strange Story of False Hair*, 1971.
Nater and de Groot, *Survey of Surveys*: 1985.
Ames, Kammen & Yamasaki, 'Hair Dyes are Mutagenic,' *Nat. Acad. Sci*, USA, Vol. 72, June 1975.
Castle, Charles, *Model Girl*, 1977.

9. SMALL IS BEAUTIFUL: THE FEET

Levy, Howard S., *Chinese Footbinding*, 1966.
Chang, *The Chinese Gentry*, (extract from Univ. of Washington Publications on Asia), 1955.
Rossi, W. A., *Sex Life of the Foot and Shoe*, 1977.

Rudofsky, B., *The Unfashionable Human Body*, 1972.
Extract, *Jnl of American Medical Assocn*, 1971.
Clarke, May, *Trouble with Feet*, 1969.

10. THE PSYCHOLOGY OF BEAUTY

Garland, Madge, *The Changing Face of Beauty*, 1957.
Liggett, J., *The Human Face*, 1974.
Newton, Eric, *The Meaning of Beauty*, 1950.
Frumkin, Robert M., 'Visual Aphrodisiacs', Article in *Sexology* 20, 1954.
Hume, David, *Essays: Moral, Political and Literary*, 1875.
Clark, Kenneth, *Feminine Beauty*, 1980.

11. THE REASONS WHY

Lewis, David, *Loving and Loathing*, 1985.
Cantril, Hadley, *The 'Why' of Man's Experience*, 1950.
Keenan, Brigid, *The Women We Wanted to Look Like*, 1977.
Goffman, Erving, *The Presentation of Self in Everyday Life*, 1959.
Menninger, Karl A., *The Human Mind*, 1946.
Rubinstein, Helena, *My Life for Beauty*, 1965.
Rogers, Carl, *Client-Centred Therapy*, 1951.
Stubbes, Philip, *Anatomy of Abuses*, 1583.
Gardiner, James, *Gaby Deslys*, 1986.
United Nations, *Demographic Yearbook*, 1983.

PICTURE SOURCES

Frontispiece   Elaborate body scarring: Zefa
pages 8/9   School of beauty, c. 1800: by courtesy of the Board of Trustees of the Victoria & Albert Museum

1. STARVING FOR STYLE

page 15   Model girl: Frank Horne/Rex Features
page 17   Maria Callas: Hulton Deutsch collection
page 19   The 'Ideal Woman': The Telegraph Colour Library
page 23   Female body builder: Claus Andersen/The Telegraph Colour Library
page 27   Marilyn Monroe: Kobal Collection
page 28   Shirley Rutherford: S & G Press Agency
page 31   Cher: E J Camp/Retna Pictures Ltd
page 32   Foot's Bath Cabinet: advertisement in *Illustrated London News*

2. THE BEWILDERING BOSOM

page 34   Medieval iron corset: by courtesy of the Board of Trustees of the Victoria & Albert Museum
page 37   Jayne Mansfield: Hulton Deutsch Collection
page 39   Minoan lady: Ashmolean Museum (copy of original figurine in Heraklion Museum)
page 41   Twiggy: Hulton Deutsch Collection

3. DRESSED TO KILL

page 44   Mona Lisa advertisement: Foster 2 Jeans, Paris
page 47   Don Carlos: Kunsthistorisches Museum, Vienna
page 48   Madame Dowding's Corsets: advertisement in *Society*, 1899
page 53   Bustle fashion pictures: *Harper's Bazaar*, 1887
page 53   Bustle framework: Mansell Collection
page 55   Burmese woman with neck rings: Bruno Barbey/Magnum
page 57   Tattooed civil servant, Michael Kickham O'Farrell: Mark Jones
page 59   All over tattoo: Dennis Cockell
page 61   James Dean: Kobal Collection
page 62   Male cosmetics: *Unique* magazine, styled by Iain R. Webb, photo by Mark Lewis

4. THE FACE: CHANGING THE COLOUR

5. THE FACE: CHANGING THE TEXTURE

6. THE FACE: PERSUASIVE PARTS

7. THE FACE: CHANGING THE SHAPE

INDEX

(Illustration pages are given in italic)